LIFESAVING GRATITUDE

How Gratitude Helped Me
Beat Stage IV Cancer

BUNNY TERRY

Dedication Page

To Johanna, who gave up part of her life to save mine.
To Nolan, who kept my dreams of survival alive.
And to my parents, Kenneth and Betty Terry, who
taught me every day what true faith and gratitude mean.

Acknowledgments

⌁⟶

This book began on my laptop and in a little red notebook on a red couch in a rental near the Railyard in Santa Fe. The final edit has taken place not far from there, but there have been eight years and a million miles in between, and what seems like hundreds of people who read drafts, offered suggestions and edits, and who never stopped encouraging and believing in me. You all know who you are.

In an attempt to recognize those kind souls (and in great fear of leaving anyone out, because you were all essential to the final product), here's a start.

First, to the cancer patients everywhere who inspired me to keep moving forward. To the survivors and to those who have ended their journey in their own inspiring ways; to those still traveling along this road that no one wants to travel: There is always hope. You are all about hope.

To the early readers who kindly waded through the drivel and still thought it was worth pursuing: Johanna Medina, Betty and Kenneth Terry, Belinda Andrews, Kyla Turner, Peggy Poling, Judy Robertson, Amy Sheridan, Shelley Wallin, Glena Henry, Sabrina Colson, Lauren McMonagle, and Elissa Dente.

To the editors who made my words make sense: Marilyn Abraham, Lois Swaggerty, and Libbye Morris.

To the Writing by Writers Group, who are all better writers than I am and who all read the earliest, worst, longest, and most boring version of this book and then graciously let me know how to make it better: Nancy Parshall, Anna Baker, Rebecca Allen, and Emily Weinstein.

To the writers who encouraged me: Pam Houston who patiently workshopped this book, Doug Preston who offered encouragement, Hampton Sides who offered to be an early reader. The generosity of these very accomplished writers is amazing and unexpected.

To my colleagues at Launch My Book: Joel and Laura, Jessica and Leah.

To Price Pritchett, author of *You2* and my coach, who taught me all about Quantum Leaps and who wrote the book that inspired me to keep looking for the simplest way to success.

To Zach and Lesley, who gave me two perfect reasons for staying healthy in Nolan and Jake. And to Leasa Medina, who helped get Baby Milo here just in time for publication.

And finally, to my great love, my husband Toby, who believes in every wild idea I've ever had. You are better than any dream I could have dreamed for my life.

Table of Contents

Preface

~~→

This is not the book I wanted to write. The book I wanted to write was a piece of fiction based loosely on the life I planned to live after I got through an ugly breakup and moved to Santa Fe. My heroine was going to be a woman in her early 50's, someone charming, smart, bitingly funny at times and occasionally sexy. She would be dumped in the ugliest manner possible by the much younger boyfriend she knew she shouldn't date, and desperate to reclaim her life, she would move to the city of her dreams.

That's the book I wanted to write. It would be funny and sad, walking the narrow precipice between comedy and tragedy that is the life of most of the women I know. I wanted my heroine to finally find either true love or total peace, and maybe even both.

But then I got cancer. Bad cancer. Not just a lump, "let us biopsy that to see what it means" kind of cancer, but "you have a mass in your colon that has metastasized to your liver and we hope it's treatable" kind of cancer. The kind of diagnosis that makes you bow your head to hide your tears when you hear about it happening to someone you love.

I stubbornly continued writing that novel for a couple of months after my diagnosis while my brain still functioned. I kept writing as I started chemo and a treatment regimen that eventually fogged up my thoughts and took all the words away. On the side, I journaled about what was happening in my everyday life.

I made a promise to myself and my eternally optimistic dad that I would try every day to remember at least one thing I was grateful for. Some days I felt so fearful I couldn't journal. I would write the gratitude piece on a receipt or a Post-It Note as I headed to a medical appointment or to see a client. It was all I could manage. After a while, it started to feel essential.

In the middle of treatment, someone gave me a copy of *Tattoos on The Heart* by Father Gregory Boyle, the founder of Homeboy Industries, the world's largest gang intervention program. In the introduction Boyle says, "I suppose I've tried to write this book for a decade." He talks about storing tales in his head, some of which he shared occasionally during mass, but none of which he wrote down. And then he says, "After recently bumping heads with cancer, I started to feel that death actually might *not* make an exception in my case."

Just like Boyle, I finally accepted that I wasn't getting out of this alive. I knew something somewhere would get me, despite my early certainty that I would beat all odds and live forever. I realized my stories about cancer and fear and gratitude would be lost. Someone out there who might have benefited from my scary, funny, and surprisingly positive experience wouldn't have this particular story to give them hope.

I was bummed. I knew there was a better book in my head. Or at least a book that didn't contain so many trips to doctors and needles and CT scans and chemicals. So much fear and uncertainty. So much fatigue and hair loss and lying awake nights with my brain full of unanswered questions and trying hard to see the silver lining. There had to be a better book than this one.

But Kierkegaard said you have to hear your cue. And Auden said "You owe it to all of us to get on with what you're good at."

I heard my cue. This book is those journal entries, all written during the year that cancer held my life in its hands. When I looked back, I found the major theme was gratitude; the realization that despite feeling like jumping off a building, I chose the gratitude route. It seems to have worked. It might just be the one thing I'm good at.

Just one more thing (there's always just one more thing, isn't there?). This book is my story, but it's also the story of everyone out there who's facing a bad diagnosis today, who's going to their first chemo treatment, who's talking to their surgeon about possibilities, who's considering palliative care rather than continuing their journey. This is a story of real people who deserve real hope. I know a lot of those people. Here's to those folks.

"Someone I loved once gave me a box full of darkness.
It took me years to understand that this too, was a gift."
— **Mary Oliver**

CHAPTER 1

Damn Hormones and Blind Dates

∿➤

It's the day before I'm diagnosed with stage IV colon cancer. I'm going on a blind date. This should be a sign. "You're going on a blind date? Isn't fifty-one old enough to know better? Are you a hopeless optimist or just masochistic? What other bad thing might happen this week?"

I'm the queen of getting set up. I've never been the tall, beautiful, or alluring female in my circle of friends. But after someone meets me, they decide maybe I'm a good conversationalist, and on a few occasions, the most interesting. They start creating a list of the guys they think might like me. Surely, they think, setting their friends up with a nice girl like me will end in happily ever after.

Are blind dates even called that anymore? And did anyone ever start a day that had a blind date at the end thinking, "I can hardly wait! This is going to be so much fun."

It's a beautiful November Thursday in Santa Fe. Instead of the blind date ahead, I'm thinking about Thanksgiving and how I wish my son and his wife, who were married in Austin last month, would come to visit. I have such a sweet house close to downtown. We could walk to the plaza and Canyon Road. I want my new daughter-in-law to love New Mexico the way I do.

I'm trying to remember to be grateful. Be grateful that I have friends who still want to set me up. Be grateful that I'm not in a bad relationship anymore. Be grateful that I now get to live in Santa Fe, the place I've wanted to live since I was six years old. That I'm healthy, that my kids are healthy, that I have clients I like who let me write and market for a living.

My friend, Sherry, is determined to get me out for an evening with an artist friend of hers. Everyone in Santa Fe has an artist friend. Sherry's is a guy named Binx. I swear. You couldn't make that name up. Maybe he's like a lot of people who move to Santa Fe and then change their names. I once met a woman named Thrine, who I'm pretty sure was Catherine in her previous Midwestern life.

I suspect someone named Bunny shouldn't cast stones in this direction. It's just that I'm not looking forward to my blind date with Binx. I'm going because I love Sherry, my old friend from my paralegal days, from the years when both our boys played with Legos in the bedroom while we drank wine on my Albuquerque patio.

According to Sherry, Binx is supposedly smart, interesting, talented, and sitting on a large stash of cash from selling a business doing something connected with a hedge fund. That makes him not only an artist, but a guy who might pay for dinner.

In September, I cancelled because I had a better offer: drinks with my girlfriends at Del Charro. In October, Binx cancelled, and Sherry let slip that it was probably because he had gone back to his Jemez Pueblo girlfriend, a young woman who convinced him that her medicine man said Binx had to buy her an expensive pair of Luchesse boots if the relationship was going to work. He did it. He bought her the new boots.

I wish I were the type of girl who could dream up a medicine man and get an $800 pair of Luchesse boots. I've always wanted my own pair of Luchesses. I love that story. I'm a Quay

County girl from small-town New Mexico, and it would never occur to me to make a demand like that.

I have agreed, via many texts but not one single phone call, to meet Binx tonight for drinks. I wish men still called. Phone calls seem to have fallen out of favor. It would be refreshing to have just one conversation in which I hear a man's voice before I agree to sit across the table from him.

I have misgivings. The last blind date I went on was almost four years ago, before I moved to Santa Fe. I was living in my hometown—Logan, population 1,100, a tiny place out on the plains in northeastern New Mexico. A waitress at the Annex Bar and Grill stopped at my table one night. "That hot guy in the baseball cap wants to have supper with you." In Logan, the evening meal is supper. Dinner is at noon. I love where I grew up, but you are in a different world when you're there.

"Who is that guy?" I asked, trying to get a good look at what was under the cap. First of all, why was he wearing a cap at the table? That's against the rules in my farm family. And where did he come from?

"He's been working here for a while, out at the natural gas plant. Maybe from West Texas?"

Despite the cap-wearing at the table, I let Kim, the waitress and an old high school friend, give him my card. He texted, and I agreed to meet him a couple of evenings later. The shocker came when I sat down across the table and we introduced ourselves. He was young. Too young.

"How old are you?"

"Thirty-five. How about you?"

"You are way too young to be asking me out. I'm forty-eight."

I suggested a plan to introduce him to all the eligible women his age that I knew. After a couple of months, during which we met and strategized about his love life and I listened to his stories of a broken childhood and ongoing divorce, despite the voice in my head warning me against yet another marginal choice, we started dating. I couldn't get him to pay attention to anyone else, so instead I looked at his young body and pretty face and said yes. After a year, he moved into my house.

We had some fun. We were okay together, even though thirteen years was a gaping difference in age. We had fun for three years until he decided to get another girlfriend while he was still living with me. It still stung that the girlfriend was twenty years younger than me and that they moved down the street from me. My pride had been hurt most of all, but the fact was that my last blind date had been a disaster.

He's now known as Last Boyfriend. It seems easier to avoid using his name. I spent too many months lamenting my bad judgment. It is time to regroup.

Now, despite all my best intentions, I want to cancel my meet and greet with Binx. I don't feel great. I went for a walk early in the day and had to sit down when I got to the Railyard, only a couple of blocks from my house. Out of breath. Head swimming a bit.

I'm thinner than I've ever been. Living in Santa Fe has magically blessed me with finally getting to the weight I like. My jeans are baggy. Even my skinny jeans are baggy. Getting dumped by Last Boyfriend has resulted in me finally being a size six instead of a ten on good days and a twelve on not so good days. I seem to be losing weight every day. The scale, for the first time in my life, is now my friend.

Not that I should care, right? I'm an intelligent, enlightened female. Why does it matter so much to me that I'm finally so thin?

And if I'm so thin, that must mean I'm in great shape. Why do I get so tired and dizzy on my morning walks? I've been doing a couple of miles every day for years. I'm determined to be in shape when I'm eighty. I presume I'll be alone in my old age due to my inability to find a man I can stand for the long haul. I don't want my kids to have to take care of me so I walk every day. Sometimes I run as well, although the altitude in Santa Fe has been killing me. I'm always breathless and light-headed.

The breathlessness dogged me when I went to Austin last week for my friend Jeanne's annual Halloween party. We were introduced by Two Casitas Wendy, Two Casitas being her short-term rental management company. Wendy is one of my favorite clients and she's lived in Santa Fe since she arrived in a VW Bug in 1974. Jeanne and I have become good friends, going with Wendy to the Wine and Chile Festival, hanging out at Jeanne's vacation home in the foothills off Hyde Park Road, eating on patios all over town. She owns successful birthing centers in Austin and is an anomaly, a blend of wealthy, smart businesswoman and old hippy chick midwife, appearing to be type A and sharp-edged on the outside. When Jeanne starts talking about breathing deeply and water births and catching babies, you know exactly where her heart is.

She's just broken up with a man she recognized as being mean as a snake after seven years. He used to handle her online presence, but now that he's been dumped, I'm the official writer/marketing consultant for the birthing centers. She's one of ten clients for whom I do the same thing. It's a sweet gig for me, and Jeanne's a good client.

The Halloween party was big, with more than two hundred guests in costumes invading Jeanne's house and lush backyard. When she mentioned it to me, I jumped on the chance to attend. My social life in Santa Fe is comfortable but quiet. I have the Wine-Drinking Bible Study Girls on Monday nights and the old guys and sports on TV at Del Charro several other nights a week. Wendy calls from time to time, but I don't have one specific person I see on a regular basis. Sometimes I go three or four days without running into or talking to anyone I know. Going to Austin for a party sounded like a social event I could embrace.

And it was. There was prep, which involved running all over town chasing down patio heaters and serving dishes and utensils and chairs and tables. There was hanging orange lights in the trees. At one point, I found myself at the top of a very tall ladder with a strand of lights and a hook and Jeanne below me saying, "Just a little bit higher — see that branch in the middle?" I leaned my head back and braced myself against the top of the ladder with an elbow, and the world went slightly black for a second.

I came back to myself almost immediately, but I was hot and flushed and more than a bit unsettled. "I think I have to get down for a minute, Jeanne. This looking up and reaching is making me a bit dizzy."

"Damn hormones," I muttered under my breath.

Someone from the Austin Ski Club showed up about that time and took over. I crawled down off my perch, wondering why the hell I was so damned dizzy all the time.

But then I forgot it in the flurry of the party. I wore my customary "devil with a blue dress on" costume, but this year, it was a short little blue sweater dress from Victoria's Secret, hugging my newly thin body and showing just the tiniest bit of cleavage, because that's all I have — the tiniest bit. I watched the crowd. Surely, I could meet one guy in Austin, just for fun. I didn't want anything serious. I just wanted to reassure myself that there were possibilities.

And then, there he was, dressed just like a Quay County guy. Stiffly starched Wranglers, ostrich-skin cowboy boots, sky-blue button-down shirt, and a belt with a roping buckle from some competition. He looked like home to me. I eventually stood next to him in the potluck line and said, "You know, if you weren't with that cute brunette, I'd totally hit on you."

"Oh, but I'm not! We're just really good friends. I'll introduce you to her, and she can tell you herself," he sputtered. I spent the rest of the evening dancing with this cute cowboy, thinking of future weekends on the ranch, where his sweet little mama would fall as deeply in love with me as he was going to.

Except that I learned at the end of the evening that he, too, was in costume. He was a factory worker in Round Rock, not a team roper. Not that I cared a lot; it was just a silly dream of mine that someday I might meet a guy who was just like the guys from home. Without the NRA membership but with the tight Wranglers.

Despite all the fun, the thing I noticed all weekend, in the preparation and the setup and the dancing with the cute young pseudo cowboy, was that I was slightly off. Going up and down the stairs from the patio into the backyard or walking up South Congress the next night with Jeanne or getting through the airport, everything seemed to take a bit more effort than before. I had always been high energy, but suddenly I felt like I might be coming down with something I couldn't quite put my finger on.

There was a moment on Sunday when we were sitting around the kitchen, Jeanne, her best friend Pharr who was becoming my friend as well, sweet Mary McLean, and me. Fun Austin women who sometimes came to Santa Fe. Jeanne laughed and said, "Look at Bunny. Dancing with the fake cowboy totally wore her out. She's pale as a ghost!"

Now, a week and a half later, when I shower late in the day for my meet and greet with Binx, and try to blow-dry my hair, I know I'm on the verge of some serious stomach funk. I'm dizzy, and my gut aches. A couple of days ago when I was in Logan visiting, everyone had the stomach flu. Now I think I may have it. I want to cancel the date with Binx because I feel crappy. In fact, I want to cancel it just because it sounds so damn silly to go to drinks with a guy named Binx. Bunny and Binx. Good grief.

But I have cancelled once, and he has cancelled once, and honestly, at some point, I have to agree with the world to try to date again. Not just dancing with a young hottie at a party, but really dating. I can't figure out why I would date anyone after Last Boyfriend's defection and betrayal only ten months ago, but it's high time I started acting like he didn't have any effect on me. Even my kids are starting to ask me when I'm going to date again.

I get out of the shower and go through my grooming routine. Hair gel, eye cream, and moisturizer. Not much makeup because this is, after all, Santa Fe where all the women I know look naturally amazing all the time. Maybe a smidge of mascara. Then hair drying, except that now the stomachache is worse. I'm sure Binx will suggest appetizers, and I'm going to have to pretend I'm fine.

I blow dry in pieces. When I toss my head upside down so that I can dry the hair at the back of my neck, I feel dizzy enough that I'm forced to stop for a while and lie down. *This is asinine*, I think, *I just need to text him and let him know I can't make it.* But I'm as sick of putting this off as I am physically sick.

I doubt that I'm going to be more attractive to him than a young Jemez girl with a medicine man, but at least I'll have done something to please Sherry, who has wondered about my love life recently. "There is no love life to worry about," I say, but she insists that this guy is great, smart, on the verge of fabulous. We'll see. We shall see.

It's November cool out, chilly enough that I find my fleece and throw it over my arm. Getting my hair dry was tricky. I'm hoping this is the twenty-four-hour stomach flu and not the four-day version. Four days of feeling like this would not be cool. I have things to do, new clients to see, money to make. My favorite couple in the world is coming for the weekend. There are Lava Lamps to drink at the Cowgirl.

I park in the Eldorado Hotel parking garage. I am determined to have a snack and a short conversation with this man and get it over with. I have worn my black skinny jeans, which fit just like normal jeans now, and a black top and a bright turquoise scarf. I want to pull out all the stops and try the old tricks, just to see if I can — and wearing a bright turquoise scarf is an old trick. It makes my blue eyes look nearly fluorescent.

He is waiting in the front room of the Agave Lounge, sitting on a couch beside a low table. He looks a lot like men my age — missing some hair and very thin. Men my age are either rather heavy or very thin, and I have a hard time knowing which I like. There's something a bit edgy and mean-spirited about the thinness, or at least there was before I was one of the thin people. Santa Fe is a city of very thin people, and the thin guys are always saying something like, "You look great. You must work out." Not, "You look really smart. Read a lot of books?" which is what I want someone to say to me. If someone would just use that line, I might fall in love on the spot.

He's also wearing a dangling blue bead of an earring. I am immediately put off. Despite my image of myself as smart and urbane, I still tend to look at guys from a Quay County viewpoint. I know that this guy wearing this marble earring would never work at home. I could never introduce him to my brothers. Throw in the fact that he's from the northwest, some sort of a writer or artist now that the hedge-fund money is in the bank, and I almost head for the door. But after all the supreme effort getting my damn hair dry, I decide I am By Gawd going to have at least one decent drink before I leave.

It isn't horrid, but it isn't fabulous. He is sweet and smart. The earring is distracting, but I sit on his right side and spend a lot of time looking at the artwork and sipping my drink. We talk about my kids and his stepson. We eat from three plates of appetizers, one of which is Kobe beef tacos. That makes me smile. In Quay County we are always making fun of people who order Kobe beef this or Kobe beef that. The ranchers I know can't believe people want to eat beef that's been massaged and fed cold beer while they're trying to convince themselves that it's worth the extra $16 per pound.

There is one moment when we're talking about living in Santa Fe, and he says, "So, have you found any restaurants you like yet?"

I'm surprised. I'm an eater. I love food, which is why getting so thin is such a surprising bonus. Santa Fe is the dream city for food lovers. I immediately flash on La Choza's chile rellenos and Del Charro's carne adovada and that thing they do at La Casa Sena with the roasted green chile stuffed with mashed potatoes covered in cheese.

"Um, yeah, I have," I say slowly, "In fact, I have yet to find a restaurant I don't like here." It's true. I also flash on breakfast at Tia Sophia and the Pantry and Tecolote, the butternut squash casserole at the Cowgirl, the green chile huevos at Horseman's Haven. I've made it my goal to search out the best of everything smothered in green chile while living here. I'm only partially through my list.

But thinking about all this food is making my stomach lurch a bit. My side aches like I've been on a four-mile run, and I'm feeling a bit lightheaded. I think how impossible it would be to date a guy long term who didn't think Santa Fe had the best food in the world.

After about forty-five minutes of talking and eating and slowly sipping, I start to think it's time to let this one go. Like maybe I've been cordial enough and I need to be home in bed nursing my stomach flu. He protests when I say I need to leave, but when I make up a story saying I might have contracted food poisoning in the past couple of days, he takes the check and says, "Go on. I'll get this. And maybe we can see each other again?"

I don't say no. We share a quick hug, and he gives me a cheek kiss, but by this time I'm wondering how it will go when

I get to my car and need to drive home. I feel awful. Between the Kobe beef taco and the one and a half martinis and my aching stomach, I'm wondering if I might pass out just walking to my car.

But I'm a Quay County girl. I'm tough as a boot, I tell myself. A little stomach flu is *not* going to get me down. And neither is a questionable date with a guy with a blue marble earring.

CHAPTER 2

I'd Have to Be Two People

⌇➤

I'm a New Mexico native. I love where I live, so much that I write a blog titled "I Love New Mexico." I throw the word "love" around a lot. Some folks view my constant optimism as unrealistic. Pollyanna-ish. For years, I felt apologetic about it. I'd read Anne Tyler or Pam Houston and think, "Why can't I be a more serious writer? Why can't I be a literary genius?"

Then I'd sit down to write something, and I couldn't help myself. Even when my cancer diagnosis was years away, I knew to cherish the moments in my life. As Natalie Goldberg said in *Long Quiet Highway*, "Every moment is enormous, and it is all we have." When I read that decades ago, I immediately wrote it down in the brown leather address book I carried when we all still had address books rather than our cell phones storing pertinent information. I read it so often that it became my daily affirmation. When I'd consider pushing the grocery cart up to the sidewalk and wedging it there rather than returning it to the store or the cart corral, I'd remember that every moment was enormous, and if my putting the cart in the wrong place made the cart guy cranky, I'd just wasted my one moment. If I had the choice of calling my sister rather than finishing a memo for my attorney boss, I'd take that one moment to make the call. Most days, anyway.

When my kids were little and I was single and tired and broke, I'd remind myself that the dishes could wait another hour but reading a story to my daughter Johanna couldn't. I wasn't always cheerful about it. Just conscious.

Not that I was perfect. Or even particularly likable. I just worked hard at being aware of how I was spending my moments. At some point, I stopped writing my notes in the address book because it was getting filled with notes rather than phone numbers. Instead, I started carrying a small spiral notepad. I approached every day using my parents' relentless gratitude as an example, even when I was doing things like sneaking everything I owned out of a bad boyfriend's house into a horse trailer parked at the curb. I'd write *Grateful for I don't have to deal with that kind of crazy anymore, happy Johanna will be going to a better school up in the Heights, glad to be paying for my own electricity, glad to get Puff the kitty into a house with no dog. Glad to be sleeping alone again/no more having to listen to snoring. Every moment is enormous.*

While most of my friends in Albuquerque were moaning about their miserable relationships with their parents, I was trying to emulate mine. Every day was an adventure to them. My dad was always thinking ahead to the next possibility. It looked like a good way to spend a life. He was certainly the most satisfied person I knew. He treated life like a gift. So did my mom.

My mom and dad were each the youngest of ten children whose parents found their way to Quay County in northeastern New Mexico in 1914. My Grandpa Terry traded two mules and $18 for forty acres that someone else had homesteaded. The first owner found the eastern New Mexico wind and winter and relentless sun and lack of rain too much, but not Grandpa Terry. He moved his family into a half dugout on the creek-banks near Porter, New Mexico, and went to work plowing next year's crop. My Uncle L. E., number eight of ten children, was born in that half dugout. By the time my daddy came along, they had moved into a frame house.

My mom's dad, Grandpa Ayres, came to New Mexico sometime before 1920 in a wagon with his wife and three small children. By the time my mother was born in 1936, he had moved his family into a four-room house along the highway that runs between Logan and San Jon. Grandma Ayres always wanted us to know that it wasn't a highway when they first moved there and that "Mr. Ayres," as she called her husband, was the head of the Works Project Administration road crew that built the road during the thirties.

During the Dust Bowl and the subsequent Depression, neighbors loaded up and left eastern New Mexico and headed to the promised land of California. But not my family. "We just hunkered down and took care of each other," Grandma Ayres said. She didn't talk about the day when the Department of Agriculture came out and shot every head of cattle on the farm. She didn't talk about the time Grandpa fell off the windmill and broke both ankles and the young boys had to take over all the chores. What she talked about was how it felt to have her family around the table on Sunday afternoon, how every time she got up from having a baby, she and Mr. Ayres wished they had had twins.

"We like to starved to death," my Granny Terry would say. She was more direct than Grandma Ayres. "And just about the time we dug out from the Depression, although we never really got over it, World War II came along, and my three oldest boys all went off to fight."

I came from hearty stock: grandmas who hauled water from the well, who scooped sand into five-gallon buckets at the end of each day during the Dust Bowl, women who killed rattlesnakes with shovels when they found them on the back porch. My mother grew up with her Uncle Thomas Jefferson Ayres sleeping on a cot in the living room and jumping under the kitchen table to hide when the noise got too much. He had been gassed in the trenches in World War I and was silent until the moment when he would have a flashback. Then he'd yell and see things no one else in the household could see. "Just let him be," Grandma Ayres would say, and they'd work around him, careful to respect his fear.

It wasn't grim, according to any of them. Neither my parents nor my grandparents made it sound like anything other than safe and secure and happy. It wasn't easy but it wasn't grim.

I had that hearty stock in my lineage and I had Kenneth and Betty Terry for parents.

"If things were any better, I'd have to be two people." Those are the words I heard every day from my daddy. I heard him say that when I was four years old and we had moved from a tiny trailer house to an almost equally tiny farmhouse in San Jon to a tiny farmhouse in Logan where he planned to make a living as a dryland farmer. I heard them again when I was thirteen and the bank was taking the farm, and he and my mom were thinking about buying a café/ truck stop in town.

"We've hardly ever even been inside a café to eat, Kenneth," my mother said, "so who do we think we are that we can *run* one?" She wasn't afraid, just curious. She had the same faith as Dad that everything would somehow work out. They did it anyway. The Fireside Café became legend in that part of the state. Truckers from across the country stopped in so that they could visit with Dad and eat a slice of Mom's fresh apple pie.

He said it when I was a headstrong senior in high school, spending my Saturday nights in a cove out at Ute lake, drinking beer and driving fast; when I was a pregnant, unmarried college student; when I got my second and third divorces. Even when I was diagnosed with cancer. Every day of his life, my dad spoke the words that told the rest of the world that he couldn't believe his good fortune, that his life was full and blessed and happy. "If things were any better, I'd have to be two people."

Words matter. I didn't always know how much. In the beginning, I assumed that everyone had someone like Kenneth Terry in their life, someone who spoke into being what they knew in their hearts. There were thousands of days in his life when his outward circumstances didn't look like what he was expressing, but that didn't keep him from saying it.

Today experts call this an affirmation. For me, it was just my daddy talking.

It was a gift to grow up with those constant words of gratitude. At eighty-eight, he still uses this language, along with words of praise for his entire family. He makes a list every morning. In the middle of the list it says, "Tell Betty how perfect she is," or "Give Betty a kiss," as though he still needs to remind himself. By example, he taught me to do the same. At some point in my adult life, I began to make the daily list of what I cherished most, along with what I needed to accomplish that day.

What I didn't know was that this practice would help save my life.

After the blind date with Last Boyfriend and the blind date with the blue marble earring, I wrote almost the same thing: *Thanks for dinner paid for, for unexpected conversation, that I'm not still married to an alcoholic.* I wasn't grateful for every facet of the evening, but I was grateful for being able to come up with something. Somehow, I knew that if my life were any better, I'd have to be two people. Even if I was feeling rotten.

CHAPTER 3

Passing Out in the Soup Aisle

∿➤

This night is not good. In fact, it's beyond bad. I pride myself on being healthy and never sick. I always tell people I stay healthy because I'm on my own. There's no one to hold my hair when I puke, so I've made a life decision to never be sick. If I have a cold, I take echinacea and drink hot water with vinegar and honey, and I get myself over it by sheer will.

Being sick is not an option. Ever. And because I don't allow myself to think about being sick very often, that's how it works out.

But I am sick tonight. Really sick. Sort of frighteningly sick. I don't throw up, but I am up and down and going to the bathroom every hour or two, waiting for something dramatic to happen. It doesn't. My stomach feels like it's on fire. Turning on my left side helps a bit, but not much. I try to think about what I have in the house. Pepto-Bismol? I always liked that the last half of that name reminds me of abysmal. You have to be feeling that way before you want to subject yourself to the pink stuff. Tums? I try both, and get slight relief, but what I keep waiting for is the urge to throw up so that I'll feel better afterward. I finally treat myself to an over-the-counter sleep aid, thinking rest will be the best thing for whatever ails me.

I still have the floors to clean and the sheets to change and some blogs to write in the morning. Sabrina and Bruce will be here on Saturday. I have to get better.

Sabrina is one of my oldest friends. She is part of a circle of old friends and adopted family. I'm excited to spend a weekend with her and her sweetie.

I sleep for a while, and when I wake, I can hear the ding, ding, ding of the crossing signals for the 5:15 a.m. Railrunner headed to Albuquerque. The sound makes me feel better, and I get up and touch my stomach and think that I may be on the mend. Sleeping for three hours straight may have worked.

I have a list of things to do. I've created a new website for my content management business, and I need to update the About page. I need to write a blog post for Wendy at Two Casitas and one for Pick Up Sticks. And those damn floors are calling my name.

I try to drink coffee, but it doesn't taste right. I sit at the computer and compose something for Wendy about Christmas activities at the Palace of the Governors. She also needs five hundred words of random copy about Santa Fe. I'm determined to churn that out, although I don't feel inspired after my short night. I look at the Pick Up Sticks editorial calendar. Yes, I can do this. Yes, I can, yes, I can.

I'm better, I think. I come from the old school of "get up, wash your face, and see if you feel like going to work" instead of lying in bed and moaning. That was always my rule with my kids when they complained and wanted to stay home from school. They had to get up and see how they felt after a shower. It was how I was raised. If you felt sick, it had better be serious before you could waste a day in bed.

I write, I post for my clients on Facebook and Twitter, and I check a couple of LinkedIn profiles. While I'm working, I think about the floors. I will start in the entryway with the painted hardwoods. It's the first thing guests see, and it's the easiest to clean. Sabrina and Bruce are not coming until tomorrow, so if I tackle it this morning and do the brick floors this afternoon, I can run a mop over the rest of the hardwood floors early tomorrow morning, and I'll be done.

I get out the mop and the Murphy's Oil Soap and carry it all into the front room of my 1928 adobe bungalow. This house is much more expensive than anything I should be renting, but it is charming and quintessentially Santa Fe, with a long front portal and the only picket fence on the block. When I was looking at houses, I told myself I wanted a true Santa Fe experience. I might go broke in the process, but I wanted to know if my dream to live in Santa Fe was the real deal.

And, of course, I had to have a house that my friends would want to visit. After my self-indulgent six months of being pathetic after Last Boyfriend, I wanted everyone to take one look at me and say, "She has really got it going on." I suspect I am still my high-school-girl self on the inside. I want to let everyone know I'm making it big, even if I'm not.

As I squirt the Murphy's Oil Soap on the floor and mop it up, I'm trying to think about how much I love my life instead of how tired I am. *I will not be sick. I will not be sick.* I have a fun weekend planned and I've already received a text from last night's date. Although I'm sure I'm not crazy about him, the attention is nice.

"Is it too soon to tell you I had a great time?" he texts. I smile. How would it be to date a guy who paid attention and made me feel like a million bucks, even one with a silly earring? "Not too soon," I text back. "Very busy today, but I had a good time, too."

That should do for a while. I don't have time to get into a textathon with blue-earring guy, but I don't want to be rude. Maybe at some point, I'll work on liking him. Or someone. It irritates me that he doesn't call. When did we stop picking up the phone and hearing one another's voice in this world? *Texting is too easy*, I think.

What I do have time for is mopping the floor. But I'm so tired. I sit down for a minute and think about what I have in the pantry that will make me feel better. Campbell's chicken noodle soup was my mom's go-to comfort food when we were home sick from school. She made delicious homemade soup, but being farm kids, it was a treat to get store-bought. Campbell's chicken noodle soup and chocolate pudding were my sick-girl favorites, and suddenly I have a longing for both, neither of which are in my pantry.

I leave the mop bucket where it is and drive to Albertsons at De Vargas Center. My stomach is still acting the double ass, feeling hot and tender and keeping me right on the edge of nauseated. There is a relentless ache in my right side. I know that the chicken noodle soup will make me feel better.

At Albertsons, I head for the soup aisle. But first I find the crackers. I can't have chicken noodle soup without crackers. And because the crackers are closer to the baking aisle, I find a box of chocolate pudding. I'll make myself the ultimate Mom meal, even though my mom isn't here to make it for me. I wish she were here. I am truly feeling like shit.

With a bag containing only saltine crackers and a box of Jell-O instant pudding, I find the soup. I'm seriously light-headed. When I add two cans of chicken noodle soup to the bag, I feel a wave of dizziness. The bag is simply too heavy. I sit down on the floor of Albertsons in the soup aisle on a Friday morning, wondering what the hell is going on, while I put my head between my knees and try not to throw up. This is shaping up to be a humdinger of a bout of stomach flu. All I want to do is go home. All I want is a tall glass of ice to chew on. I know that would make me feel better immediately. But I don't have the energy to get over to the deli section, where they have fountain drinks and ice. For some reason, chewing ice makes me feel better these days. It's my new addiction.

Instead, I make myself get up and go to the cash registers and wait patiently in the express lane. In the car, I call Jeanne in Austin. She's the only medical person I can think of.

I describe my symptoms. "Bunny, you sound really weak," she says. "I think you need to go to urgent care. I think you might have appendicitis or a gallbladder issue."

"I can't have either of those. I cancelled my health insurance nine months ago." I curse Last Boyfriend for deserting me with a pile of bills in January, leaving me unable to afford my self-pay health insurance. How does a grown woman get to a place where she has no health insurance? Good grief. I should have sold some plasma. Anything to keep my health insurance. But I was healthy and I had never used it for more than an annual exam, so why keep paying $375 a month for it?

"How much could a visit to urgent care cost?"

"Probably a hundred bucks," I say, thinking of my bank account that is nice and fat right now with my house-sale money, funds I don't want to use for medical expenses.

"Well, good grief, you're trying to pass out at Albertsons," Jeanne says. "I don't think a hundred dollars at urgent care is going to break the bank. You just don't sound like yourself. You have to go."

I think of my beautiful bed in my comfy little house, of making myself a can of soup, of getting the floor mopped and things picked up for Sabrina and Bruce. I think of what fun we're going to have tomorrow, and I know that I don't want to be laid up for any amount of time.

But Jeanne is right. I probably need medicine to make this go away and get better. I have $100 to pay the urgent care bill, even if I would rather spend it on the hand-embroidered tunic I saw last week down at Parts Unknown near the plaza.

I go home, unload my incredibly heavy bag of groceries, consider pouring out the mop water, and instead get online to find an urgent care. The problem with being new in town is that I don't have a doctor. In Logan, I'd go to the clinic and get a shot, and the drama would be over. I hate drama.

And until this moment, I've forgotten that I'm supposed to go to Mu Du Noodles tonight with Charlotte and her pal, Trish. Charlotte is a new friend, someone I met at the Cowgirl. She called me early in the week, and I was invited into her circle of Friday night dinner friends. I was excited that we were going to Mu Du, which is supposed to be elegant and delicious. If the urgent care doctor says I have something more serious than the stomach flu, I'm going to miss out on dinner.

Dammit. I hate to be sick. I want to have dinner at Mu Du.

But I do what Jeanne says. I locate an urgent care with good Yelp reviews and I take my pathetic self to the clinic on Rodeo Road. This is when I miss having a boyfriend. Some guy I trust should be helping me into the car, making sure I'm comfortable, glancing sideways at me to be sure I haven't passed out. He should drive me there and anxiously wait with me. But I don't have a boyfriend or a spouse or anyone who's particularly worried about me except for Jeanne, who has made me promise I'll call her the minute I see the doctor.

There is the requisite filling out of forms, the signing of documents that says yes, I know, I'm a self-pay, I have no insurance; yes, here's my debit card, and you can charge me the $114 for an office visit. It's not breaking the bank, but it's not getting me that tunic from Parts Unknown, either.

There is a wait. It's November, the season of babies with fevers and little kids with deep coughs and runny noses. I wait about forty-five minutes and feel progressively weaker until I almost fall asleep in the waiting room before my name is called. I've downloaded *Pride and Prejudice* onto my Kindle app, and I'm through the part where Elizabeth meets Mr. Darcy before they call me back.

I'm weighed, and even on a doctor's scale, I'm proud to see I'm down to a weight I haven't seen since my second divorce.

That one left me very thin. I have a tiny moment of elation. Since January 1 of this year, when I was left high and dry by Last Boyfriend, I have lost a total of twenty-two pounds. Even in my dreary state, I wish he could see me now, and I wish I could snub him and say, "See! See how much better off I am without you?"

Instead, I'm ushered into a room where the nurse takes my vitals. "Your blood pressure is a bit low," she says, "eighty-five over sixty."

"That's normal for me," I tell her. "I always have low blood pressure."

She shakes her head. "Most people's blood pressure goes up when they go to a doctor."

I don't care at this point. I just want someone to take a quick look, give me some medicine, and usher me out the door to my fun weekend—Mu Du Noodles and Saturday with good friends.

The doctor is young and sweet. He looks like he's about twenty-two, the age my daughter Johanna will be in a few weeks. He tells me I'm running a low fever and I have that low blood pressure, and could I lie back and let him examine me more fully? He puts his hands, one over the top of the other, on my stomach and begins pushing and probing. When he gets to the right side, where I've indicated I have some discomfort, and pushes hard, I want to come off the table and slap him.

"Ouch! That hurts," I tell him.

"It's also hot," he says, "and I think you may have an appendix that needs to come out."

I groan. I don't have time for an appendectomy or anything of the sort. But he is insistent that I need to go to the emergency room, and he wants to call an ambulance.

I say no. Yes, I have $114 for this office visit, and I have money in the bank from selling my house, enough for an ER visit, but I sure as hell don't want to waste cash on an ambulance run. And there are all those little kids in the waiting room. Wouldn't it frighten them to see me go out on a stretcher?

"I'll drive myself," I tell him.

"The weather's starting to get ugly out there. That rain's supposed to turn to snow. You sure you're up for driving? You know where the hospital is?"

I have a vague recollection of the location. I tell him yes, and when he says, "We're both adults here. You know that you have to pull over if you start to feel dizzy, and you have to call an ambulance," I nod, climb off the examining table, and find my way to the car.

Before I start the car, I call Johanna's cell phone. I'm too tired to drive and talk on the phone at the same time. It's 3:00 on a Friday afternoon by now. She'll probably be on a court run for the Albuquerque law office where she works when she's not in class. I suspect she won't answer her phone. I'm right. I call her office instead and get the receptionist, who promises to pass along a message.

"Please be sure she gets it," I say. "Tell her I'm on my way to the ER at St. Vincent's. The doc thinks I have appendicitis."

There is immediate concern in her voice. "Do you need me to send someone to the courthouse to find her?" she asks.

"No. Don't scare her. Just have her give me a call when she gets this."

There really is no reason to call Johanna. It is just preferable to calling my parents, who are in their eighties and would immediately jump in the car to make the three-hour drive. And there is no one else who needs to know.

Then I call Sherry. She texted me earlier and wanted to know about my date with Binx. I can give her that information and tell her I'm on my way to the ER. It probably won't be anything. I think I'll be home in a couple of hours. I'm still hoping for Mu Du Noodles.

"I've been dying to hear from you all day," Sherry says when she picks up the call. "How did it go?"

"It was fine," I tell her. "He was what you said. Nice and smart."

"You don't sound very excited. In fact, you don't sound good at all."

I tell her about feeling crappy and the urgent care visit, and I tell her I'm on my way to the ER.

"Oh my God," Sherry says. "I'll meet you there."

I try to tell her it's not necessary, this will be quick, surely there is nothing very wrong with me, but that now I have to get on the road. My gut is aching. Maybe I just need to lie down for a bit.

At St. Vincent, they get me right into an exam room, and a nurse shows up in minutes. "Let's check your vitals," she says, a very cute, hippy chick with dreads. I smile. *I'm not going to have an operation, I'm not going to have an operation, I'm not going to have an operation*, I say to myself over and over. I'm convinced of the power of positive thinking. How else have I gotten where I am? Living my dream life in Santa Fe with a dinner date with a group of interesting women. A man who bought me not one but two drinks last night, even if I didn't drink the second one. A job where I get to work from home. A bit of a cushion of cash in the bank, which is new in my life. I am *not* going to have an operation.

Maybe I have an ulcer, although I think that requires a personality that frets. I am not a fretter. Maybe I ate bad bagged salad. Maybe I have an ectopic pregnancy. I almost make myself laugh with that one. *You have to have sex to get pregnant*, I say to myself, *and you, my dear, definitely have not had sex in a really long time.*

"Wow! Your blood pressure is seventy over thirty. How are you walking upright?" Cute nurse with Nicki on her name tag looks worried. "Let me get our doc in here."

It's an icebox in the emergency room. Why the constant cold? Something about germs? Despite the chill, I am, as always, craving a bit of ice. I think they bring you ice in the hospital, although the last time I was in a hospital was when Johanna was born in 1990. I'll have to ask Nicki when she returns.

An older (my age) bearded doctor comes in. He pokes around and makes noises about my low blood pressure and slight fever. I assure him that just by making me lie down, the hospital has probably cured me. There is talk of an ultrasound and blood work to see if there's anything weird going on, and Nicki comes back with an IV kit.

"Do I really have to have an IV?" I ask, knowing that this is just another cost I'll have to pay out of pocket.

"Those are the rules," Dr. B says, and Nicki nods.

"I'm really good at this," she says. "You won't even know I've poked you."

I don't mind the poking. I mind the wasted cash and the fact that it's getting later and later in the day, and my Mu Du Noodle dates need to be informed. I text Charlotte with an "I may not make dinner tonight. So sorry" message, thinking that I really want to get to know these women better, and cancelling on them will not be good form.

Sherry shows up, breathless from the cold outside. "It's trying to snow," she tells me and then wants the rundown.

"It's not a big deal. I already feel better," I tell her, "This was a silly idea, coming to the ER. Let's talk about my pseudo date instead."

"He really likes you," she says. "I can tell by the way he told me about last night. I don't think he thinks it's a pseudo date."

I settle in for postgame analysis. This is really the only reason to go on dates—so you can talk to your girlfriends about them the next day. Dating is a total drag, and I'm not good at it, only because I hate the follow-up. I like the anticipation, the possibility that I might be about to meet someone who will totally get me *and* know how to two-step and quote Shakespeare while shaving. I love the idea of dating and romance and true love. What I don't love is the reality, the sifting, the settling, and most of all the disappointment.

I tell Sherry that I liked Binx fine and that he's already texted me today to suggest that we do it again. "See, I told you he likes you!" she says in that excited high school voice women sometimes use with each other when they're discussing men.

"We'll see," I tell her. "He's a bit intense. And he said the one thing that totally threw me off."

"What's that?"

"He asked me if I had yet to find a restaurant in Santa Fe that I liked."

"What?" she asks, laughing. "How crazy is that?"

"Yeah, I know. I have yet to find a restaurant in Santa Fe that I *don't* like. Have you?"

"No," she says, shaking her head. But she's immediately back on how I can fix that, how he's from Seattle, how he just needs to be educated, and if anyone can lead a non-native to a good time and great food, it's me. Except that I'm done with fixing anyone. I've proven myself a total failure at that over and over.

Nicki shows up with a wheelchair. "We're taking you to the ultrasound room," she tells me, and we leave Sherry behind with her visions of me showing Binx how to be a true New Mexican.

CHAPTER 4

Craving Ice and Eating Raw Meat

~~→

It's now 7:30 p.m. I've officially missed my Charlotte/Mu Du dinner, and I'm hungry. The last thing I ate was half of a Kobe beef taco at Agave last night with Binx, and I didn't eat a lot of that.

Johanna is here with her current beau in tow. Sherry has headed home to Albuquerque in the sleet and snow, me shooing her away with an assurance that I'll soon be home.

We're all bored, and the doctor comes in to say that the ultrasound didn't really show anything. "Stand up for me and walk heel to toe," he instructs. I do that trick, and he probes my stomach one more time.

"I don't think this is your appendix," he says. "I'm going to send you home right after we get your blood work done. You feel better, right?"

I do feel better. Just lying down and being still and resting, which are three things I seldom do other than late at night, have made me feel better. There is a dull ache in my side, but it's nothing dire. It feels a bit like a menstrual cramp, which I haven't had in eighteen months. Probably my damn hormones. Or lack thereof.

I'm embarrassed. Johanna and Jason have come up for the evening instead of staying in Albuquerque and doing whatever college students do on a Friday night. There is nothing substantially wrong with me, and we're all sitting in a small, cold room watching bad television while we wait for blood-test results. Jason eventually goes back to my house to let Lucy the Pug out and get something to eat. I'm instructed not to eat until they know what's up, and I'm already planning what we'll pick up on our way home. A chile relleno burrito from the Burrito Spot sounds delicious right now. A green chile cheeseburger from Blake's. Anything.

But then Dr. B is back, frowning over a clipboard.

"Where's all your blood going?" he asks.

"What do you mean?"

"Well, something's going on here. Your hemoglobin is 5.2. If you were a trauma patient coming in with this count, you'd be dead."

I frown. There is nothing wrong with me and no reason for me to be anemic. "Well, I've been out of breath a lot lately," I tell him.

"Do you have any weird cravings?" he asks.

"Does chewing ice count?"

He nods his head. "Absolutely. How long have you been doing that?"

Johanna rolls her eyes. "She chews ice all the time. It's a little crazy how much ice she chews. And annoying."

"And when did this start?" Dr. B asks.

I think back. It may have started right after Last Boyfriend left, but I chalked that up to nervousness. And there's another craving I've had that I'm not going to mention to him.

Back in December last year, T. J., Robin, and I decided to split a half of beef from a grass-fed beef ranch up at Nara Visa. The bulk of it was ground beef, but there were a few roasts and steaks. For months this past spring, my thoughts all day were on all that red meat in my freezer, and I would go home to a piece I had carefully thawed the night before. And I would eat it raw. It was delicious, this organic, grass-fed beef with no additives.

I've never told a soul, and I'm not about to tell this guy. That's probably what's made me sick. I'm probably suffering from something really ugly, like worms, from eating raw meat.

There's a moment when everyone leaves my cubicle in the ER except for Johanna. We look at each other.

"Mom, what's going on?" she asks, her eyes wide.

I don't know the answer.

And then there's another doctor with us. He introduces himself as the attending physician on call. He speaks slowly, or I hear it slowly, or I don't hear it at all. At least I'm not sure I understand everything he says.

"We're going to admit you, my dear, because it appears you may have a mass on your colon."

I hear it as *mess*, his East Indian accent confusing in the fluorescent glare on this late Friday night. I have a mess in my colon. That's not a big deal, right?

Okay, so what's next, I ask, and he responds that I'm going to be moved upstairs where I'll get prepped for a colonoscopy. Not a big deal, I think again. I've never had one before, but so what. Right?

I have my first colonoscopy the next afternoon. I want instead to be at the Cowgirl BBQ drinking a Lava Lamp with Sabrina and Bruce. That had been the original plan. A Lava Lamp is Pabst Blue Ribbon beer mixed with a swirl of frozen margarita, which makes for a delicious way to spend a Saturday afternoon.

Instead, I am dressed in a gray hospital gown lying on my side while the nurse explains the twilight drug that will "help with any discomfort." Gray is not my color, and to add insult to injury, a tech is threading a scope with a camera into my intestine by way of my rectum.

It has been almost exactly twenty-four hours since I drove myself to Urgent Care at Jeanne's suggestion. There has been the inevitable waiting that seems to go with being hospitalized. By 3:00 p.m., Johanna, my parents who drove up early this morning, Sabrina and Bruce who showed up anyway, and especially me, are all tired of each other and ready to get the scan over. I am starving, ready for a green chile-smothered burrito at the Pantry Café.

I send everyone away, telling them to go find lunch. Before they leave, my mom insists that we all join hands and pray that God's hand is on me, that the scan will be quick and painless. She also prays for peace for all of us.

I wish she would have prayed for me not to be hungry. I am so hungry. I am feeling better. I want to go home. At some point during the day, I checked my little red notebook where I had a long list of things I needed to do. I wrote a couple of things I was grateful for: *Jeanne for making me see doc, that Mom and Dad made it here safely.* Usually I write five things I'm grateful for. It's an old practice, almost a rule. But today, waiting to eat and for my tests to be finished, I am delirious thinking about that burrito. I'm surprisingly not worried. I just can't think of many things that make me feel grateful today.

Instead of getting a burrito, I get a drug in my IV that makes me groggy. I already received four pints of blood in the past twenty-four hours that made me immediately feel better than I have felt in months. Amazingly my ice craving has disappeared. I had no idea I was so tired.

This new IV drug, like the blood, is doing whatever job it's supposed to do. I'm relaxed and feel like my head is wrapped in cotton. Here's that peace my mom asked for. No nervousness, not even when the nurse asks for my daughter's cell number so they can have my family in the waiting room when the scan is over.

A tall, striking brunette enters in a white coat and introduces herself.

"Where are you from?" I ask from my fog, thinking maybe I hear an accent.

"Portugal," she says, waving her hand as if my question is a pesky gnat.

She has me shift slightly to my left, indicating the screen above my shoulder, and says, "If you stay awake, you can watch with us. Now we will see what is going on." I feel light pressure and then see images of what I always thought my esophagus might look like. But this is not my esophagus.

"Aha!" she says. I am startled by her voice, but glad I am so relaxed. "There it is! See that?"

On the high left-hand screen on the monitor, she points out a fleshy, angry growth of something that looks like a dark pile of meat gone bad in the fridge, pulsing with energy. "That's cancer! I've been doing this for seventeen years, and I know cancer when I see it."

I close my eyes, hoping this is a nightmare. It has to be. Any minute, I know I will wake up on the patio of the Cowgirl BBQ with a Lava Lamp in my hand, Sabrina leaning across the table to tell me a juicy bit of hometown gossip. Any minute.

CHAPTER 5

Movie Cancer vs. Reality

⟋⟍⟶

I know almost nothing about cancer, other than what I've seen in movies and read in books. I was a sophomore in high school in 1976 when my Uncle Lewis died a slow and painful death from throat and lung cancer. As sick as he was, he worked hard to be cheerful when I was around, except for that moment when he grabbed me by the collar and pulled me close. "You *ever* put a cigarette in your mouth, and I'll come back to haunt you!" He was more emphatic than I'd ever seen him. Otherwise, he was his quiet self, continuing to watch out for my Aunt Mattie while he slowly wasted away. I cried for days when he died.

And I've never put a cigarette in my mouth. Thank you for that, Uncle Lewis.

In the '70s, cancer movies were a genre of their own. *Brian's Song*, an ABC Movie of the Week, was one of my favorites. It was agonizingly beautiful, ending when former Chicago Bears player, Brian Piccolo, played by the very handsome James Caan, died from cancer. His best friend, Gayle Sayers, played by the equally handsome Billy Dee Williams, was slowly overwhelmed with clarity and goodness while he watched Piccolo waste away. We all cried around our high school lockers the next day talking about it.

Cancer was so sad. But it was so illuminating. It made for great stories.

Ali McGraw in *Love Story* was the epitome of beautiful and smart and the woman we all wanted to be when I was in junior high. So what if she had to die at the end? She still got to talk like a sailor, using language that my parents and uncles discussed at the supper table. They'd never heard anyone use the "F" word in a movie before. She had Ryan O'Neal renouncing his fortune for her.

There was *Terms of Endearment* and *Beaches*. Everything I learned about cancer, other than what I knew from my Uncle Lewis, I learned from television or at the Odeon Theater in Tucumcari.

From the movies I'd seen as an adolescent, it looked like cancer had the potential to be moving and healing in an emotional but not physical way. And then you died. I couldn't recall any movies that involved the star of the show going through the brutality of treatments and hospitalizations and surgery who then got well. There didn't seem to be any inspiration in getting well.

I also knew nothing about the staging of cancer, other than when Laura Linley yelled into the phone on the HBO series *The Big C*. Her insurance company put her on hold once and she shouted, "Don't put me on hold, dammit! I have stage four cancer! There is no stage five!"

My second night in the hospital, after the colonoscopy, when I still didn't know for sure what was going on with me medically, I wrote in my notebook: *Glad I finished the blog posts for Pick Up Sticks, happy Sabrina still came to town even if I can't go shopping, excited for Ambien prescription and sleep.* I didn't say anything about what the gastro doc had told me during the screening. I didn't feel grateful for much, but I knew I needed to write something down.

On my third day in the hospital, I thought of all those movies. When the oncologist on call came into my room that Sunday and sat down at the end of the bed, I thought of what the gastroenterologist had said during my colonoscopy the day before. I thought of her telling my parents and Johanna that I had a tumor in my colon and one on my liver.

"And we have no idea whether these are treatable or not," she said.

I thought of Ali MacGraw in *Love Story* and silently lamented the fact that I was single and in charge of my own financial wellbeing. There was no Ryan O'Neal in my life offering to fly me to Paris, or even to pay the electric bill when it came due.

While the oncologist glanced through the papers he held, my daughter sat on the bed with me, my parents sat on my right side in uncomfortable chairs, and Sabrina sat in a chair on my left, furiously taking notes. My phone was on the bed, my son Zachary tuned in by speakerphone from Texas.

Sabrina had volunteered to be the scribe, but I knew she wanted to be anywhere other than in that room. She bent over her notepad, her mass of blonde hair falling over her face so that I couldn't see her expression.

"Do you live alone?" was the first thing the doctor said after introducing himself.

I said yes, and he frowned. I was proud to be living alone in Santa Fe, finally having extracted myself from a stupid relationship. Obviously, the oncologist didn't feel that my living alone was optimal. Until the day before, it had seemed perfect to me.

He leaned forward and put his hand on my foot. "You have stage four colon cancer. You have a 5.5-centimeter tumor in your ascending colon that has perforated your colon wall. You were bleeding out with the blood seeping into your abdomen, so that's why you've been feeling a bit lightheaded. You also have a 4.5-centimeter tumor on your liver."

I still knew nothing about cancer. I looked at the tablet in Sabrina's lap. It was wet with tears. I thought of Laura Linley yelling into that phone.

There is no stage five. That seemed to mean that I had the absolute worst cancer diagnosis in existence.

There's something misleading about cancer in the movies. First, the actors are more attractive than everyone else. They live in nice homes, and money is never discussed. The doctors are organized, and everything is pretty and clean. Everyone must have insurance because there's no scrambling to be sure a procedure is covered.

Instead there's a lot of quietly discussing the future. There are epiphanies. There are long, soulful looks where the characters realize how precious life is, how important it is to set aside grievances, discussions about how to make up for lost time. There are tearful goodbyes.

On that Sunday in November, I didn't see my life as a movie version of anything.

There was a moment after the oncologist left when I heard my dad greeting my cousin, T. J., in the hallway outside the door.

"Kenneth," T. J. said with a catch in his voice, "how the heck are you?"

My dad, predictable as always, said, "Well, T. J., you know, even with all this, if my life were any better, I'd have to be two people."

Everyone in the hallway was silent for a few seconds. If anyone else had said it, no one would believe it. But this was Kenneth Terry, and all the cousins and my close friends outside my door knew that Dad meant it. My friend, Courtney, told me later that she cried when he said it because it was so true for him and for all of us. He believed we were all still blessed, regardless of what life was offering at the moment.

Then I heard a pat on the back and knew that T. J., my big burly bear of a cousin who is like a brother to me, was hugging my dad and patting him on the back. Only Dad could say that at a time like this.

I thought, *He's right. Even though I have cancer and even though my life doesn't feel like a Hollywood movie, look at these people who are here, look at my daughter sitting on the bed with me, look at this city where I get to live, hopefully for a long time. Surely if life was any better, I'd have to be two people.*

CHAPTER 6

64 First Cousins

∿➤

I was diagnosed and met my oncologist on a Sunday. That afternoon my Amarillo friend Suzanne called. I love hearing from Suzanne, but I didn't pick up. I couldn't handle one more phone call. She was one of dozens. She left a message, suggesting I start a CaringBridge site where I could post updates about my progress. "It's a great way for people to check in without having to bother you," she said. "And people will want to know how you're doing."

I am from a small town. I know everyone in my county and most of New Mexico. I have sixty-four first cousins. When I go to the State Fair, I run into twelve of my oldest friends. Three will be cousins. My circle is big. CaringBridge is a great idea.

What I'll write on CaringBridge for all those cousins and people who want to hear from me will be upbeat and chatty. But the truth will be a bit more like how I felt that first day, talking to the oncologist, and then that night at home alone, after I was released from the hospital. The only thing I will know with any certainty is that despite how I'm feeling most days, I have to write down what I'm grateful for. And I need to let everyone know that I'm fine.

I will write later, *Glad I was still pooping*, since the oncologist had explained that my colon was narrowing due to the size of the tumor. It was probably time to start praying for a miracle. Instead, my racing mind latched onto not having any health insurance, about how it seemed logical to stop paying my premiums in February when I was so broke.

I had paid for that coverage for so long, never using it other than for an annual exam, which I had every October. I was healthy, fit and thin, and I slept well. I exercised and didn't eat processed food. And, and, and, *and*...I was only fifty-one. I had this huge, exciting Santa Fe life in front of me. I had followed all the rules.

Except that I had no health insurance and stage IV colon cancer. Once again, I wondered how a grown woman who was so proud of taking back her life had no health insurance. How did someone who was so healthy and had no symptoms have stage IV colon cancer?

"There's a standard treatment plan we'll go over when I see you again on Tuesday." Dr. L had said in the hospital. "We can talk about it in more detail in my office, but it will involve chemotherapy and then, if you're a candidate, surgery to remove the tumors."

If you're a candidate. That sounded ominous, as though there was a chance that I might not be the right person to beat this. To survive.

"And we'll want to order a PET scan immediately," he said. "Since you don't have insurance, will you be paying cash for these tests?"

Earlier that morning, I had had a conversation with T. J. about the New Mexico uninsured pool. Evidently, if you have a pre-existing condition, the state has a pool that you can get into to obtain coverage. T.J. also used words like, "if you qualify" when we talked about it.

"I think I'll have coverage soon, through the state pool," I said, and Dr. L nodded.

"You'll want to check on that immediately. We'll hold off on the more expensive procedures until you know for sure."

I had just been diagnosed with stage IV cancer, and my biggest worry was what it might cost. Not an obstruction, not even death. I was most concerned about the cost.

Dr. L was clear that we couldn't wait too long on treatment. The pain I felt in my side was from the perforation in my colon wall and the pending obstruction, which could happen any day. "We don't want to have to do emergency surgery to open you up. That's risky." He explained as gently as possible that I had an open, oozing sore inside my body. It wasn't going to get any smaller without intervention.

We discussed my appointment with him on Tuesday. "I've made space to meet with you," he said, alerting me to the fact that getting a quick appointment with him might be a big deal. "Let's not talk any more about treatment until then."

It was the middle of the night when I started my CaringBridge posts. I was at home, released from the hospital. I sat down to write, after hours of trying unsuccessfully to sleep, even with a new prescription for Ambien. There was nothing to do but write it down.

In the red notebook I wrote *Glad I liked my doctor, glad to be home, glad to see everyone, glad they got home safely,* and then I stopped. I couldn't think of a fifth thing I was glad about. Instead, I went to CaringBridge and created an account. This is part of what I wrote:

> I sat on the edge of the tub tonight and cried great, wracking sobs, heaving and moaning sobs, "Why me, why me, why me" sorts of sobs that, had someone heard me, would have brought them running to see what was wrong. But no one came running because I was alone. I had sent them all home, those people who love me and who came to see me today in the hospital and then came back to the house with me afterward. Old friends and family. Johanna, my parents, T. J. and Robin and Russ,

Kene and Amy and Courtney, even my old Albuquerque pal, Bruce Davis.

Stage IV, the doctor said today. All we knew was that there wasn't a stage V.

My cousin Jennifer and Mari Anne Ban, my pastor's wife, came by the hospital earlier, bearing a hand-knitted prayer shawl from my church's shawl ministry. I remember thinking several weeks ago how I would love to have one of those shawls, and how it was too bad you couldn't just purchase one because certainly I would never have a reason to need one.

It was a day filled with friends and family and love and care and good wishes and a lot of tears and then finally, a late lunch at the Pantry with fourteen of us at the table after I was finally released from the hospital.

It was odd to me to be at the center of it, to be the one sitting on the bed. I am always the first one to show up at a hospital when someone's admitted. I'm the one willing to drive great distances to offer comfort if you or your dad or your mom or your husband has gotten the bad diagnosis or is in the next room dying. I'm the one willing to go for cafeteria coffee or sit with you in the waiting room while you wait for the surgery to be over.

I was raised by people who did the same, who treated it like an honor, their Christian and civic duty, folks who did it without question or complaint. We're good in a hospital room. We show up, smiling, bearing magazines or flowers or candy, or coloring books if that's what's warranted.

Today was the first time I was the reason people showed up, and it was also the day an oncologist turned to me and said, "You have stage four colon cancer, along with a 4.5-centimeter lesion on your liver. Your lymph nodes appear to be involved as well."

Here's how my life has been until last Thursday: I finally live in Santa Fe, where I've always wanted to live. I live in a 1928 adobe house with great vibes and wood and brick floors and tongue-in-groove ceilings and a wood-burning stove and a wide portal in front and a patio out back with a coyote fence. I even have a true tin roof, something from my childhood dreams.

I walk to the Plaza or to the Railyard, to the Cowgirl or Second Street Brewery. I go out to dinner with friends, flirt with bartenders, field a few calls, and think about going on dates. I have a group of adorable men in their seventies and eighties who shout, "Hey, Bunny from Logan!" when I walk through the door of Del Charro. We watch baseball and drink beer together a couple of nights a week.

I write a lot, mostly for other people to make money and to handle their social media accounts, but also the novel I plan to finish this year. I try to make at least one new friend a week. It works. I like this life. In fact, I love this new life in Santa Fe.

So today. That was different. Dr. L, my new oncologist, said, "You're a medical anomaly. You have no genetic tendency to colon cancer, you're fit, you're under sixty, you're female, you've never smoked…according to the stats, you shouldn't have this."

I am not writing this post to get sympathy. I have a plan. No more sitting on the edge of the tub, crying about something that I can't change with tears. No more wondering why me, and why my kids and why my parents. Why isn't important.

If I have to assign a reason to it, let it be this: I'm going to do this, and I'm going to do it well, and I'm going to write it all down to make sense of it for someone else. I'm going to make a road map of my journey. I'm going to continue to be grateful, even if there doesn't seem to be anything to be grateful about. This may be a journey worth recording if it helps someone else do what I want to do.

I'm going to kick cancer's ass. Sooner rather than later. Thanks for checking in.

CHAPTER 7

Don't Get on the Internet

∿➤

Monday. It is the first day after my diagnosis. I woke up this morning automatically thinking about traveling to Logan this week to work at the real estate office. I'm still a partner there and when I moved to Santa Fe, I promised to put in at least two days a week. Then I remembered.

I have cancer. I remembered the pain on Friday and the evening at the ER and the colonoscopy and the throbbing, angry mass on the screen in the scan room. That's why my side hurts. That's why I'm taking hydrocodone, as much as I want, according to Dr. L. No limits. No admonitions about possible addiction. Later I will write in the red notebook, *Grateful for pain meds.*

I think of all the calls I've already received. It seems like hundreds. Even on silent, my phone buzzes every few minutes. Everyone wants to talk to me and reassure me of their prayers and care and love. Or maybe they want to reassure themselves. Regardless of the reason, my phone rings nonstop. I'm choosing not to answer it.

I'm standing in front of my desk, where I would normally sit down and check on a blog post for one of my clients, respond to comments on Facebook, or compose the day's tweets. I look at my computer. Dr. L said a thing that was repeated by my day nurse and again by Laura, a nurse friend who goes to my church.

"Don't get on the internet," they all said. Dr. L said it very quietly. "I'd suggest you try to keep yourself from getting on the internet. It will only make things harder."

But this is what I do. I am on my computer all day long, locating or disseminating information or curating content. Surely just one look won't hurt.

I log on. While my computer is loading, I get another call from a sort of friend, but more of an acquaintance. I feel guilty, but this is just one more person I can't stand to talk to today. He was really Last Boyfriend's friend, and when Last Boyfriend went south on me, Vince became my friend. *News travels fast in Quay County*, I'm thinking. Vince must already know I have cancer. He's a sweet guy who has seen me through a hard time. I don't answer. I can't talk to another person right this minute.

I'm getting on the internet.

I type in "stage IV colon cancer." The first organic site is cancer.org, which sounds like something legitimate. There is a listing that starts with stage I, then II, then III. Stage IV says that my cancer is one that "has spread from the colon to distant organs and tissues." I don't think anything in my body is very distant from anything else, but okay. What else? What did I not hear Dr. L say?

The site says, "In most cases, surgery is not likely to cure stage IV cancers." Wait! What? Surgery worked with my brother-in-law. He's cured. But what stage did he have? And what stage did his brother have, the one who died from this disease? Oh, hell, why did I have to remember that Richard died from colon cancer?

I am steadily more confused and distressed, but I read on. There is a statement that says if your doctor recommends surgery, you should know whether it is to "cure the disease or simply relieve your symptoms." I read about a colectomy, where they remove your colon above the site of the tumor and reconnect it, sometimes requiring you to wear a colostomy bag, which is a bag where your waste is collected outside your body. Oh dear. That never crossed my mind.

I go back to Google and look at other pages. Cancer Treatment Centers of America says, "The stage of colorectal cancer is one of the most important factors in evaluating treatment options." Yes, I know. I have stage IV. There is no stage V.

This site also says there is a commonly used staging system called TNM, which looks at whether your cancer involved a tumor, lymph nodes, or metastasis. My understanding is that I have all three.

There are supposedly Cancer Treatment Centers of America everywhere, so I click on the Locations button. Atlanta, Chicago, Phoenix, Tulsa, Philadelphia, Seattle—none of these is a place I want to think about going today.

I'm clicking back to Google when my phone rings again. It's my sister, Belinda. I know I can't avoid talking to her. And it's okay. She's already been through this with her brother-in-law, Richard, who died from this disease, and her husband, Andy, who had surgery and survived. This probably upsets her more than almost anyone. The odds should have been in her favor that another member of her family wouldn't get colon cancer. Sorry, sister.

"Hi, sistah," I say in my brightest Monday-after-cancer-diagnosis voice. "How are you this morning?"

"Well, I'm fine. I'm calling to check on you." Her voice is a bit breathy, like she's trying to temper whatever it is that she wants to say. Or she doesn't want to cry. I'm really making folks cry these days, it seems. She lives in Lubbock, and I know she wanted to be here yesterday. We all seem to think we should gather in whatever hospital a family member finds themselves. She missed the drama and the chance to comfort me in person.

"I'm okay. Still have cancer this morning," I say and then think, *what a smart-aleck asshole I may become during the course of this illness.*

"That's why I'm calling. Kyla and I have been talking. We want to pay for you to go to Phoenix to the Mayo Clinic for a second opinion." Kyla is my niece and Belinda's daughter. She's a Southwest Airlines employee and has flight benefits. She could get me free tickets anywhere, and now that's what Belinda is offering.

My mom had thyroid cancer almost ten years ago, while I was living in North Carolina considering slitting my wrist because my alcoholic husband was making me so crazy. No lie, but that's another story that required a lot of red-notebook entries. Thankfully, I made it home safely from that debacle.

While I was there, Mom went into the hospital with a lump in her throat that the doc and a dozen tests had sworn was benign. "We'll just operate and remove that," her doc said. "No problem."

While I was trying to hold my precarious marriage together too many miles from home, my mom went under the knife and woke up to a cancer diagnosis. I talked to my sister a lot that week. Everyone will tell you if you get cancer, thyroid is the best, as though one is better than the other. Mom ended up with an oncologist who was caring and aggressive, Dr. A from the Texas Tech Medical Group in Amarillo. Now she keeps mentioning him to me, and she's discovered that he's moved to Albuquerque to UNM Cancer Center.

I can't think of a logical reason that I don't want to go anywhere else. Conventional wisdom is that you need to get a second opinion. But what I also know is that I am over-whelmed by the mere mention of my cancer. I am paralyzed. Right now, I'm up to my ears with thinking about cancer and comfort and wanting the latter more than the former. All I can think is that it's not like another CT scan is going to make my tumors go away.

I tell Belinda I'll think about it. "I love you, Bendy," I say, "but I have to get off the phone."

I write in the red notebook, *Thanks for Bendy and Kyla.* But I don't want to go to Phoenix to the Mayo Clinic. I don't want to go to any one of the six locations of Cancer Treatment Centers of America. I don't even want to go sixty-five miles down the road to UNM for a second opinion. I want to stay home. I mostly want to go back to last week at this time when I didn't know anything about colon cancer or staging or metastasis or Dr. L or the ER at St. Vincent's Hospital. I want to be well again.

CHAPTER 8
The One Thing

~~→

It is Tuesday, the day of my first office visit to the oncologist. I don't know what to expect. I only know that he found a way to fit me into his schedule in just two days.

On Sunday in the hospital, Dr. L vaguely outlined a series of steps that we might discuss, but today I am worried that he'll suggest something drastic, like surgery next Thursday, or that I move to Phoenix to the Mayo Clinic. My family is rallying around. My niece called last night to make her sweet offer to fly me anywhere I want to go. My parents have called at least three or four times to check on me. I know they are calling aunts and cousins and their pastor and friends. It feels like a continual buzzing in my ear.

The one thing I know right now, getting ready for my 11:00 a.m. oncology appointment, is that Johanna is on her way from Albuquerque to go with me to the doctor, and my cousin Jennifer will join us there. She'll listen and take notes while I put my life in this seemingly kind man's hands. We've arranged to go by Christ Church on our way so that our pastor, Martin, can pray with us. I need to spend a minute or two with him. Martin's great gift to us is his calm assurance. He is not a pastor who raises his voice to make a point; in fact, he frequently lowers his voice when he most strongly wants to convey a message. You're sometimes forced to lean in to hear him.

I dress, feeling better now that I have these pain meds and the Ambien that helps me sleep. There still is a relentless stitch in my side, but now that I'm resting, I don't feel like I'm going to pass out. And with four new pints of blood coursing through my veins, I have no craving for ice. None. After months of chewing chunks of ice like a maniac, my higher hemoglobin number has cured me of that crazy craving. I am still relieved that I didn't develop the other craving the ER doc says sometimes accompanies low hemoglobin: eating dirt.

This morning I wrote in the red notebook, *Grateful for the new blood, Ambien, Johanna coming, doctor visit, Jennifer.* These feel like all the things that will get me through one more day.

Johanna arrives, and we try not to be testy with one another. She is as nervous as I am, which is considerable. At the church, we're greeted by the staff, including Jennifer who will follow us to the Cancer Center. And Martin, in his customary jeans and polo shirt. He looks more like a surf instructor than a pastor, which is reassuring. A traditional pastor would pray for me to be healed. I'm sure Martin will come up with something better than that.

And he does. We gather in a circle, me in the middle with Johanna, and Scooter, the sweet old guy in charge of the prayer ministry, anoints my forehead with oil, something this Baptist girl has never had done to her. And then Martin prays.

His words are simple. He doesn't start by thanking God for this opportunity to feel His good grace or by asking for a miracle of healing. What he says is, "God, we come to you today asking that you put blinders on Bunny, that you let her see only the hurdle that is directly in front of her. Help her not to look forward at whatever obstacles might or might not exist out there. Let her see only one thing at a time and let her know that she is required to do only the one thing that is right in front of her." He goes on to ask for grace for Johanna and for me, for my parents and my friends and the rest of my family.

One more time, he reminds God (and me) that the one thing I need most is peace and to find the calm in this particular storm.

It is a simple prayer, but it is the best prayer anyone has ever prayed for me. It is possibly the best prayer I have ever heard, and my brain tilts toward that idea, the idea of only trying to tackle the one thing in front of me, the next thing that has to be done. I'm pretty sure I can do this. I have spent my life racing ahead, trying to juggle a thousand ideas and thoughts, as well as activities and obligations, when all I had to do was the next one thing.

My next one thing today isn't conquering cancer or making my parents and my kids feel better. It is just to see the oncologist. That is all I have to do in the next hour. It is the only thing I have to think about. With blinders on, it is all I plan to do. Later this evening, I will write in the red notebook, *Grateful for the blinders prayer. One thing.*

CHAPTER 9

My Head Is Spinning

〰➤

We are officially on pins and needles. Jennifer
follows us from Christ Church. Johanna and I do not speak,
mostly because we are petrified. What now? What will he tell us
that he either didn't say or we didn't hear on Sunday morning
in my room at St. Vincent's? Jennifer is here to be the sane set of
ears in the room, and she carries a spiral notebook into which
she will write a lot of notes in the next several weeks. She is a
gift, moving through our lives with her calm and her beautiful
red lipstick. I really should ask her what brand she uses. It is
always perfect.

The Cancer Center is an inviting building, as inviting as a
cancer treatment facility can be. The entrance is a south-facing
wall of glass surrounded by Pueblo-style architecture. The
waiting room for the oncology clinic is tastefully decorated,
with expensive prints of locally known artists. There's a Keurig
in the corner under a large-screen TV where The Barefoot
Contessa chops something that looks like onions or jicama
and swipes it off the cutting board into a stockpot. I wish I
were home chopping onions. Jennifer senses my unease and
puts her hand over mine. I am so grateful for her.

I've checked in, writing my name on a clipboard and
marking the box that says "doctor." There are two more
boxes—one that says "treatment" and one that says "labs."

I'll learn the drill soon enough. When I come in on Wednesdays for chemo, I have to see the doctor first. But before Wednesday chemo visits, I will have to come in each Monday to have lab work done. Johanna and I will become friends with the girls in the lab, especially the cute young one from Pecos who wears red Converse Chuck Taylors every day. I'll learn to ask what the orders say because the one time they forget to have me do a urine test, I'm in trouble with my clinical trial director and have to have the test on Wednesday before they'll let me have chemo. It will become my complex dance — the tests, the blood work, the getting ready for chemo.

But I don't know any of this yet. I only know that I have a long road of unpleasant procedures in front of me, and I don't particularly want to participate. I don't even want to talk about it. I want to go back home and write a blog post for someone, something really neutral that has no bearing on anything in the world other than whether someone is buying charms or chains from Pick Up Sticks or books a house this weekend with Two Casitas. I just want to go home.

I am now done with my first oncologist visit. Johanna and I made plans for the afternoon that included queso at Junction along with a beer, but we are not there. We didn't even stop for lunch. Instead, she is in her room, which isn't her permanent space yet but will be, and I am in my room, pretending to take a nap.

My head is spinning. Thank goodness Jennifer agreed to go with us to both this appointment today and the chemo orientation this Friday. I have always prided myself on being quick and clever, but today I was plodding and slow and not clever in any way. I had no personality or energy. I knew this was a hurdle I had to get over, but I barely made it. I try to feel grateful for something. I have nothing.

There was a lot of talk about my tumor markers, which I now know are also called my CEA. In technical terms, "CEA" is carcinoembryonic antigen, a measurement of proteins associated with tumors. It's a term we'll become all too familiar with in months to come.

We discussed a PET scan and a port and X number of rounds of chemo and then perhaps surgery. The words "if I am a qualified candidate" came up again and again.

Dr. L was as kind and gentle as he was in my hospital room two days ago, but he was also purposefully vague. We went in wanting concrete answers, and instead there were discussions that focused on my insurance status.

"No, I don't have health insurance today, but I should have it by December 1," I said a couple of times, and he and the clinical trial director would consult calendars and shuffle papers. It was determined that the clinical trial would pay for me to have a quick CT scan and an EKG to be sure I'm a candidate for the trial. I want to get in the trial. I want to get whatever new drug they're trying that will attach itself to my antibodies, or maybe the new drug is an antibody, or maybe the new drug will fight antibodies. Honestly, I am so foggy on the trial, but so anxious to try anything, that I don't remember all of the details.

What I do remember is that everyone was distressed about my lack of insurance.

Dr. L told me a few concrete things: "Eat whatever you want. Beginning right now, you need to try to gain some weight."

Gain some weight. These are magical words if you're someone who's always hovered just a tiny bit over your best weight, although what woman doesn't believe she's always been slightly overweight? Even knowing now that the cancer is what caused my weight loss, I admit that I really like being a thin person for once. I can't seem to get over the thought that the thin me is just a slightly cooler version of the not-thin me.

I have cancer *and* I'm still shallow. One would have thought those two are mutually exclusive.

I want to be Dr. L's best cancer patient. Instead, I think about how much I weigh and how much this will cost.

"Get a lot of rest," he added. "You need to view your tumor as an open wound, even though you can't see it. Don't over-exert yourself."

I was not told, nor did I ask, how long I might live with stage IV colon cancer and a tumor on my liver. We did not talk prognosis. We did not talk anything other than next steps. Perhaps Martin's prayer is working. Perhaps I am getting it, and everyone else connected with my disease is, too. I can only do what is in front of me. Perhaps the doctor doesn't want to say what he thinks.

Johanna comes into my room. "I have to go back to Albuquerque for classes early tomorrow," she says, and I see how exhausted she must be. Has she slept this week? How is this going for her? I remember the day I heard that my mother had thyroid cancer, just a tiny little lump that was easy to remove, and suddenly my heart is broken all over again.

"Are you resting?" I ask. "Do you want some of my Ambien?"

"Mom, I hear crazy stories about people who take Ambien. In fact, I'm not sure you should even be driving on the days after you've taken it. And yeah, I'm sort of resting. I just have a midterm to get through this week."

Johanna will get up early tomorrow and go home to Albuquerque for her classes, and I'll stay here. Unless I can snag someone else to go with me, I'll be alone when I go for the CT scan. I'll be alone when I go for my EKG. I am fifty-one years old, and for the first time in my life, my single status terrifies me. For one, I know I will never go on a date again as long as I live, however long that might be. For another, I have no one to hold my head if I puke after chemo. I have no one to lie awake with me late at night to talk about how afraid I am. I have no one. Because your kids shouldn't have to be the people who do all of that for you.

Despite everyone's assurance that they are here for me, I am all alone in this fight. It feels so solitary, so quiet in my head, even with my racing thoughts. The only thing that makes me sane is stopping occasionally to write it down. *Grateful for Johanna being here today.* But even that feels lonely. I am so alone and so ill-equipped for this. I do not want this to be my life.

Johanna crawls up on the bed with me and asks, "But what about you? Did you rest? Are you okay? Do you want me to stay here and call my professor? I think I can say my mom has cancer and get out of my exam."

I look at her for a minute, and we both start laughing. "Holy shit!" I say. "This cancer may be a great thing if it gets you out of a midterm."

We turn toward each other, and I hold her hand in mine. It is not true that I am all alone. It is not true that I have no one. I have Johanna. And about a million other people who will help me with this. The hell with dating.

CHAPTER 10
Playing the Cancer Card

∿➤

Saturday evening after the fateful colonoscopy, my brother Kent called to see how I was doing. Kent is the sibling closest to me in age. He was five when I was born, and when the conversation around the table at family gatherings steers to our childhoods on the farm and how incredibly low on cash we were, how the boys had to start driving a tractor when they were ten and eleven, how they had to save every single penny to be able to afford their first car, Kent always says, "But not Bunny. She was the baby. She got everything she wanted." I don't quite remember it that way, but everyone has his own story. His about me is that I was indulged and adored. What I recall is that we were all adored in amazing ways.

But starting on the day we all hear about the cancer, me from the gastroenterologist and him from my mom weeping over the cell phone, he has been sweet and encouraging and, for the first time ever, quick to say "I love you" over the phone.

He called me that Saturday night in the hospital, starting with a hesitant, "Well, I guess we got some bad news today." There was a catch in his voice, but he maintained calm for as long as we were on the phone. He said all the right things — that I'm tough, that I have everyone rooting for me, that I have a lot of people on my side, an army of sorts, and after we talked a while and I was stoic and said I basically felt fine and that I was going to get better, he said, "You know, this is the same cancer that Sarah has."

Will is my brothers' childhood friend and Sarah is his sweetie. I've met her once, but Will is one of those family friends who only shows up for funerals. He likes us, generally, but his history with my family is based on when my brothers were young. Sarah is slim and pretty in that relaxed Santa Fe, no-makeup kind of way, with long, thick, curly red hair and a brusque manner that makes you think she might not like you at all. I've sent Will a text since I've been here, but I haven't pushed it. He was friends with my brothers. He and I hardly know each other.

He and Kent are close, guys who like to hunt and fish and camp out in the northern New Mexico woods away from people. He's invited Kent and Viola to his place in Chama, and when he shows up for the annual funeral we always seem to have in our family, they stand around outside together, talking construction and elk permits and Republican agendas.

To hear that Sarah has colon cancer is surprising. I'd heard through the family grapevine that she had some kind of cancer, but I assumed it was breast. What a stupid assumption, but like the rest of the world, when I hear that a female has cancer, I assume it's in the breast.

"No," Kent said, "she has colon cancer that also showed up in her liver."

Just like mine. Weird. Really weird. I asked him to give Will a call and let him know what's up with me. If I have at least a semi-ally who has been in my shoes, I may make it after all.

I hear from Will late on Tuesday after the first oncologist visit. It's a phone call instead of a text, and he's apologetic that I've been in town so long and we haven't gotten together. Then he says, "Oh, Bunny, I'm so sorry you have to go through this. It's so awful." We talk about Sarah, and she gets on the phone and she is, as expected, all business.

"Who's your oncologist?" she asks.

I tell her that Dr. L was the oncologist on call when I was in the hospital and that I just had my first appointment with him.

"Ah," she says. "He's mine as well. We kind of have a love-hate relationship, but I think he'll take good care of you. Will and I want to have you over for dinner so that we can talk to you about this and see how we can help you."

I agree to dinner and we set it up for Wednesday evening. I'm happy about this. So what if I had to get cancer to get invited to spend an evening with Will and Sarah? I have a good feeling about this.

I know where they live because I looked it up and walked past there a month ago. It's about five blocks from my house, which means that we've been silly not to be in touch before. But Sarah is battling cancer, so maybe they don't have a lot of time or inclination for visitors. I'll have to remember that tactic.

The house is on Elena Street off West San Francisco Street, which Sarah says she bought years ago when the neighborhood was sketchy and before gentrification. Will is a contractor, so everything is beautifully remodeled. Sarah has a loom in one of the bedrooms and she shows me new fabric she's woven for a jacket she's making for a juried show, where she hopes the judges will choose her design over hundreds of others

Honestly, they're far too cool for me to be hanging out with, but here I am, me with my cancer and her with hers. While Will orders takeout from Yin Yang, Sarah and I sit at the bar and she gives me a gift she's chosen especially for me. It's a three-inch, three-ring binder.

"You'll need this," she tells me. "They're going to give you piles and piles of paper, and you'll need a place to keep it all. And then they'll give you more. You're going to have to be really organized."

I'm not organized at all. And now I'm overwhelmed. But I'm grateful for her candor.

Finally, we talk about her cancer. She went in for a routine colonoscopy and was told that she had stage IV colon cancer that had metastasized in her liver. She says when she came out from under the anesthesia, Will was sitting beside the bed with tears in his eyes.

Like most people, she wanted it OUT OF THERE. Immediately. And after lots of wrangling and fighting with Dr. L and searching for a surgeon who would do it laparoscopically, she had the tumor in her colon removed. Wham, bam, thank you, ma'am. Gone.

Except that she was left with the liver lesions. And by the time she had healed from the colon surgery and could start chemo, she had numerous spots on her liver. At least that's how she explains it to me.

Now, eighteen months after her diagnosis and after months of chemo, she is on a once-a-month lifetime chemo maintenance regimen that is supposed to control the colon cancer in her liver. This is what I'm learning. Although the cancer is currently located in her liver, it is still colon cancer because that's where it originated.

Sarah is sick of cancer. She's even sicker of chemo. She's sick of what she says is the culture of cancer, the doctors who don't think outside the box, the ongoing treatment that seems to have no end, the marginal progress she's making with the chemo. She shows me her port and says, "Yeah, this is what yours will look like, and yeah, it hurts like a bitch for a few days after they put it in. But you'll get used to it. Ugly, right?"

She gives me helpful tips. I wish Johanna or Jennifer were here to take notes. "Use the lidocaine they give you. Cut a piece of Press'n Seal a few inches bigger than your port, slather it with lidocaine and press the plastic against your skin. That'll hold it until you get to the chemo suite. The needle they use is huge, and this will keep it from hurting."

Ick, I'm thinking. I've worked hard on not thinking about the mechanics of the chemo and I'm still two days out from my orientation so I don't know a lot, but Sarah knows the truth. They're going to put a mechanical device under my skin with catheters running into my veins near my heart and a large needle is going to pump chemicals into my system. Every two weeks, rain or shine.

By the time Will gets back with the Chinese food, Sarah and I are old friends. We've talked about hemorrhoids ("Listen, Bunny, when that chemo gets ready to leave your body, it will do it with a vengeance. If you don't have it already, get some Preparation H right now."); hair loss ("They'll tell you it will be minimal, but look at this pathetic ponytail. I used to have piles of hair."); and nurses ("Ohmigod avoid the crazy one at the chemo suite if you can. She's so scary!"). I'm drinking a beer which Sarah advises me to enjoy. "I can't even stand the taste anymore," she says.

Hanging out with Sarah is amazing and a relief. Yes, we have cancer, and yes, that totally sucks, but here she is, eighteen months out, walking upright, giving me sarcastic but damn funny insights, and she's surviving. Will tells me that they're going to Denver to see a doctor who plants radioactive seeds in livers that have inoperable tumors just as soon as insurance approves the procedure.

"I can't do chemo forever," Sarah says, "and that's what Dr. L wants me to do. On and on and on. At some point I have to pull the trigger and find another treatment."

I think of all the phone calls I got from Belinda and Kyla. They're still trying to get me to Phoenix to the Mayo Clinic and they're willing to foot the bill for it. I appreciate their desire to get me the best treatment, but I can't wrap my head around it at the moment. Cancer is such a looming presence in my life that I can't think about anything other than starting treatment here and seeing how it goes.

Sarah reassures me. "I totally get it," she says. "Being away from home at a time like this would be exhausting. Do what you can do here and then see what happens."

We end up in the living room, Will and Sarah on the couch, me in a very hip midcentury side chair with my feet up on their coffee table. I think once again how shitty it is that I got cancer but how cool it is that I get to hang out here.

"God, Bunny, I just hate this for you," Will says again, just like he said it on the phone. "I've been thinking all day, knowing you were coming over tonight. I've been thinking about what advice I'd give you, what I'd tell you to help you get through this. And the best thing I know, the advice I keep coming back to is this: Play the cancer card. Play it every single time you get the chance. If you have to have this in your life, you might as well use it to your advantage."

I laugh. "Honestly?"

Sarah laughs with me. "He's right, you know. Milk this for all its worth. You're going to go through some awful times, and you might as well make it worth your while. And this: When people offer to do things for you, *let them*."

It's good advice. Something I hadn't considered. I feel like I'm in a maze, stumbling through piles of information and trying to get appointments set up and worrying about money and Johanna and Zach and my parents. I didn't know there might be the slightest advantage in any of this. But Will's right. I can play the cancer card. Right now.

"Well, then, I need another beer, Will. Can you get it for me, because you know, I have cancer?"

He laughs and gets up from the couch. "Good job, Bun. I think you're going to be just fine."

CHAPTER 11

I Am Not Grateful for Cancer

~~→

People want to come and see me. Lots of people. The first weekend after I got out of the hospital, I was insistent that only Johanna was allowed. I needed a day or two with her to breathe and *not* talk about what's happening. We made a point of doing what we liked. We went to Junction for chips and queso. We went to the movies at De Vargas. We walked around the Farmer's Market, and on Sunday morning, we went to church. Church was a blur, with the folks who know about me coming up with tears in their eyes and a hug. I had lived in Santa Fe only three months, and I had been looking forward to getting to know all those Christ Church people better, but was this the way I wanted to deepen those relationships?

Until my diagnosis, Johanna was planning to go to Wisconsin in January to live with her boyfriend who is headed there to begin grad school. She wanted to try something new, and while I wasn't convinced that Jason was the guy for her, I knew that she had to figure it out on her own. The move to Wisconsin had distressed me. I knew she needed to find her own life. I just didn't want it to be so far away that I couldn't drive there if she broke an arm. Or had the flu. Or needed her mom.

On the morning after my diagnosis, Johanna climbed up on the end of my hospital bed and sat facing me. "I'm not going to go to Wisconsin, Mom," she said. "I'm going to move back to Santa Fe in December after finals and live with you while you get treatment." This was after Dr. L had looked at me with those sad brown eyes and asked, "You don't live alone, do you?"

I was grateful and heartsick at the same time. I seem to be grateful and heartsick a lot these days, but this made me especially so. I didn't want Johanna to stop being a college girl. I didn't want her to have to give up this last semester of undergrad studying and playing and enjoying her early twenties to take care of her mother who just happened to have cancer. Mostly, I didn't want her to have to be my care-taker when I had always been hers. But there it was—my living alone seemed untenable at best, and it wasn't as if I was willing to leave Santa Fe and move back to Logan to live with my parents.

So now I have Johanna staying in New Mexico. I insisted that we have one weekend to ourselves, although I knew it pained my parents and siblings and everyone else in the world to be cut off from us.

That was the first weekend. Now people are becoming a little louder in their requests to spend time with me, and in fact, I'm having a hard time saying no. I'm torn. I love my family and friends, but I hate talking, talking, talking about cancer and how I feel and what's going to happen and what the doc said and what procedure is next. I hate being treated with kid gloves.

Glena and Yvette have been here to give me a spa weekend. My cousin Janis came up for a night. Keith and Angie from

Logan dropped by to spend the night on Wednesday. Angie swore she had to see that I was still okay.

Sherry called yesterday and wanted to run by the house, but I was going to be out.

"How are you?" she asked.

I gave her the standard answer. "Fine. Sleeping better with the Ambien, taking some pain meds, anxious to get this show on the road as soon as my insurance kicks in. And how are you? How's the new paralegal gig?"

"Ohmigod, you know how lawyers are…they make things so. . .it's just such a…" and she trailed off. "Oh, it's not so bad. Certainly it's nothing like what you're going through."

This is happening a lot. I'll talk to a friend and ask how they are and they'll begin with, "Ugh, this was such a shitty day…but you know, things aren't bad at all. Not compared to what's happening to you."

I'm pretty sure they're thinking, "At least I don't have cancer."

This is just another thing I hate about having cancer. Evidently, when I was diagnosed, I immediately lost my ability to be a friend with good listening skills. No one will give me bad news or say anything honest about the marginal day they had at work. When T. J. calls to talk, I ask how things are at the office. I know the answer in November will be "too damned slow, no traffic, no new listings," et cetera. But what I get instead is, "Oh, you know, it's all good. Really good."

I know people are determined to keep things light for me because my life seems so difficult. But, really, I'd like to hear some real-world shitty stuff. It would keep me from feeling like mine is so bad.

I broke down and allowed Sabrina to come up earlier this week. She wanted a specific task and offered to clean out my pantry.

"No, not that," I said, trying to think what I might have that would be her strong point. Sabrina is not a fan of any kitchen in general unless someone else is standing at the stove doing the cooking while she drinks a beer at the bar and visits with them. "How about organizing my closets and the shelves in my bedroom? My scarves and purses are a big jumble."

My charming Santa Fe House has no closet space to speak of, so I have boxes that have been under my bed since the August move. It was the perfect chore. She not only organized my closet and emptied boxes; she went through my chests of drawers and made the space make sense. I wrote a couple of blogs, she worked, and then we met on the patio for a glass of tea. I know Sabrina is sick with worry over me; she is one of my oldest and best friends, and she has taken the stance that maybe if we don't talk about it, everything will be just fine. She says, "Don't use the 'C' word with me." When I ask whether the "C" word is cancer or chemo, she says, "Uh huh. Exactly," and goes on with her organizing.

I'm okay with that right now. Not talking about cancer is a huge favor to me at this moment. Later when it's not so new and raw, I will want her to allow me to talk about cancer, and she'll still resist. Today, I understand and I am grateful.

Other people say things like, "Let me know if there's anything I can do." What I want is for a cleaning crew to show up and say, "We're taking over. We're cleaning your house." I don't want to assign tasks, except to Sabrina, who won't mind anything I say to her as long as I don't use the words "cancer" or "chemo."

This is my best advice if someone you care about has cancer. Don't say, "Let me know if there's anything I can do." Just ask permission and then show up. Send a beautiful handmade plush blanket, like Judy from Logan did. Send an inspiring fluffy pillow, like Jill from Albuquerque did. Clean their yard. Hire window washers to only do the outside. Send a gift certificate for pizza. Do something physical or concrete that will bring comfort or make things easier, like Sabrina did.

That's what we all need. We just need more of it when we have cancer.

On Sunday night after the weekend alone with Johanna, I write in the red notebook, *Grateful for two days with my girl, queso at Junction, Alex for sending me new clients, Josh at Ranch House and Paige at Santa Fe Modern for hiring me, movie popcorn*. I should have written, *Not talking about cancer once this afternoon* because that is the gift that Johanna and I give each other. But I don't want to write the word "cancer" in my gratitude notebook. I am not grateful for cancer.

CHAPTER 12
Telling the Truth

∿➤

To appease the people who want to hear how things are, I make myself write a CaringBridge post at least once a week. The posts are sometimes sticky sweet and always optimistic. I'm writing these posts for my mom and dad, for my Aunt Jackie and Aunt Crystell, for the little old ladies in my parents' church, and for the people in my hometown. I started the posts to keep everyone informed and maybe to lessen the number of phone calls and texts I get every day.

Because there are still a lot of phone calls. People are encouraging and kind and promise to say prayers, or the ones who don't believe in prayer send me their best thoughts. Sabrina has a friend visiting Paris this week, and she posts a photo on Facebook of the candle the friend lit for me at Notre Dame. It gets eighty-three likes in the first three minutes.

I say in my first CaringBridge post that I wouldn't want anyone else to get this cancer, and that's true. But I didn't want *me* to get it, either. As soon as my insurance kicks in, I have a list of medical procedures. The one I dread the most is the port placement, where they'll cut my chest open above my collarbone and slide a piece of plastic under my skin after they've woven a tiny little catheter line through my veins (or is it arteries?) into my vena cava, whatever that is. Wikipedia calls the port a "small medical appliance."

My orientation nurse flipped open a notebook and showed us an actual port yesterday. And yes, I had to go to chemo orientation. This is a learning experience I would happily have skipped in this lifetime. The port is about half an inch thick and three-quarters of an inch in diameter. It's where the chemo will be "delivered" by a needle. I read that chemo is toxic to muscles and skin and that a port is considered the best possible method for chemo treatment.

I've seen Sarah's port. In true Sarah style, she said, "It hurts like a sonofabitch when they put it in. I'm just telling you. But you gotta have it." Hers is an unattractive bump under her skin, and I'm pretty sure mine will keep me from having sex for a long time. Not that I necessarily want to have sex this week, but at some point, I'll be interested in that sort of thing again...won't I?

I get that the port will hurt. As will the chemo needle. There. I've said it. I don't want things to hurt. I don't want to get neuropathy in my hands and feet, which is something we talked about in orientation, or extreme sensitivity to heat or cold, or nausea or diarrhea or hair loss. The technical term for hair loss is *alopecia*. Another thing I didn't need to learn in this lifetime.

Sarah has had every possible side effect from her chemo. Her feet are raw, her hair is thin, her sense of taste and appetite are nonexistent. "Don't even get me started on the diarrhea," she says. There isn't a lot of talk, either from her or the orientation nurse, about nausea, although movie cancer makes a big deal about it. Evidently, I will receive an infusion of anti-nausea meds at the beginning of each treatment. Okay. Silver lining. I'll take it.

Right now, I don't want to be the person with all these medical procedures on my calendar or any pain on the horizon. Instead of thinking about it, I write in the red notebook, *Grateful for Sarah telling me the truth, for Yin Yang Kung Pao chicken, for*

The Big Bang Theory, for Downton Abbey, for Lucy the Pug. Lucy is Johanna's dog, who has come to stay until Johanna can be here full time. We got Lucy when she was the tiniest of puppies, the runt of the litter. Johanna was a freshman in high school and Lucy spent her early days with me at the real estate office, cradled in the crook of my arm. Lucy doesn't care that I have cancer. Now at eight, and a bit chunky for her age, she just wants to lie in my lap while I watch more television than I've watched since I had mono in the eighth grade. She loves *Downton Abbey* as much as Johanna and I do.

To maintain my optimism, I write this CaringBridge post the day after my orientation:

> My dad's mantra has always been, "If my life were any better, I'd have to be two people." While I'm not thrilled that I've been diagnosed with cancer, I have to say that my cup runneth over with all the love and care and encouragement I've received in the past two days from my extended family and friends.
>
> I appreciate all your calls and texts. If I don't immediately get back to you, just remember that I'm talking to lots of medical folks and getting my ducks in a row. I'd truly love to spend my entire day on the phone hearing from each one of you, but eventually I'm going to have to get to work.
>
> Feel free to leave a note here. Will update this journal next week after doctor visit. Thanks for checking in.

What I felt like writing instead was this:

> I'm scared. I don't sleep at night unless I dose myself up with Ambien. I roll the words "stage IV colon cancer" around in my mouth, slowly saying them aloud, and wonder what it would be like to have a significant other. Johanna will be moving here permanently as soon as her

semester ends, but for now she's here on a sporadic basis. Other people want to visit all the time, but I don't feel like entertaining. I'm lonely and cranky, frightened and sometimes wishing there was a man sleeping with me, cuddling up early in the morning, brushing my hair back off my forehead, bringing me coffee in bed. Offering lots of positive support. Loving me despite my cancer.

I thought I might have found a guy I like on OkCupid. He contacted me through an old profile from this summer. We've been emailing each other for a couple of weeks. He's tall, smart, and funny, and we're working up to a meet and greet, but honestly, don't I have to tell him I have cancer? Isn't the protocol that this would be the ethical thing to do? Isn't stage IV cancer kind of a pre-first-date disclosure requirement?

There's also Clint from Kansas, a guy I met long ago at the Cowgirl. I lost his contact info and just found his email address a few weeks ago and got back in touch with him right before my diagnosis. He is wholesome, cornfed sweet. We're supposed to go out for drinks this weekend, but I'm thinking I should text him with the truth. Weird thing is that his mom died from colon cancer. I remember that little tidbit from the last time we saw each other for drinks at Pranzo in the Railyard. I like him with his sandy hair and green eyes, but I'll bet I'm no longer as interesting as I was when I was just a fit Santa Fe girl with blonde hair and blue eyes. I'm pretty sure having cancer lowers your attractiveness level considerably.

It seems unfair. A loser of a young guy ugly dumps me and when I finally get to live somewhere interesting and beautiful and potentially full of available men, I'm diagnosed with cancer. What the hell?

You have to have some huge faith to keep believing God knows what He's doing. Today, I'm not certain.

CHAPTER 13

Grace and the Wine-Drinking Bible Study Group

∿➤

The Wine-Drinking Bible Study Group has a standing Monday night dinner, but this will be the first I've attended since my diagnosis. Johanna is invited this time, and she's a bit apprehensive. "Why do I need to go, Mom?" she asks. She's twenty-one and not excited in any way about spending an evening with a bunch of church women. I get it.

I tell her I want her to meet these women and that we'll probably see a lot of them in the next few months. In October, long before anyone knew I was sick, I went to my first Bible study with them, and as I came through the door, my Southern Baptist brain was thrilled to see that there was wine on the counter. *Now, this is a Bible study I can get on board with,* I thought. *Thanks for the Wine-Drinking Bible Study Group,* I wrote that night.

I am still trying to process my situation. I can't start treatments yet because of no insurance, so the pain in my side has not subsided much. But I feel a thousand times better after the four pints of new blood. My brother, Klee, laughed on the phone and said, "What if it's Republican blood?"

"I'm pretty sure my political convictions have already converted it," I reply. We are frequently on the opposite side of the political spectrum but hearing him laugh on the phone this week rather than having a catch in his voice is an improvement. Klee, who's had a lifetime fight with an alcohol addiction, poured everything out and declared himself a non-drinker this week. It is a victory in this turmoil that is my life and we're taking wins wherever we can. He's on my side, he says, and I believe him. My family and friends are rallying.

So now Johanna and I, me with my stitch in my side but with hydrocodone working on it and making me slightly light-headed, are on our way to Lauren's. She lives on Old Santa Fe Trail near Museum Hill and St. John's College, in a neighborhood of homes that I've always wanted to visit, dreaming of living there. There are high adobe walls with gates around these properties and Lauren's is no exception.

Lauren is a pretty, blonde sprite of a girl, probably not much older than my son, Zachary. She is the mother of Johnny and Will, who are four and six, and twins, Hannah and Tate, thirteen months old. I do not know her well now, but eventually I will get to spend many evenings on her couches and back patio, drinking wine and talking. We will be an unlikely pair, but she will become one of my best friends and supporters.

I don't know that yet. I just know that I'm the sick one and there are women in this house, waiting to hover over me and check me out. I feel like I'm a science project to be gawked at. I'm probably underestimating the intentions of the people who care about me in a genuine way, but I can't help my self-consciousness.

Johanna and I pull through the gate. The house is a New Mexico midcentury adobe, the sort of place I could only dream of owning someday. Johanna parks, and we walk through the courtyard gate. Through brightly lit picture windows, I can see women moving about in the open living area and kitchen. I see someone with a wine bottle. This is going to be all right.

It is intimidating to walk into a room of women you barely know as the newly diagnosed cancer victim. There are women here I've never met — Asha, the tiny Indian girl who looks like she just finished high school, and Tyra with the dark hair and great lipstick. But there is also Mari Anne, the pastor's wife; my cousin, Jennifer, who helps us hold our world together; sweet Megan, who is Lauren's sister-in-law; Stacy with her Dallas accent; the other Jennifer, who will leave next week to go to the Galapagos to photograph wildlife for *National Geographic*; and Keadron, the art therapist. Kristi and Cristiane are here, too. This is a room filled with beautiful women who love Jesus, which in turn means that they love me. It's all grace.

They crowd around, hugging us, Mari Anne wiping away a tear. I know they mean well, and I am happy to have them in my life, but I am overwhelmed. I silently pray for more grace. Later, Lauren will tell me that she spent the entire afternoon praying and that she was apprehensive about how I would look and how I would feel, about how everyone else would behave around me. She expected Johanna and me to be sad and a bit beaten and more emotional, not bright and smiling. I didn't think about how this would be for everyone else; cancer has made me a bit self-centered. But we are fine. *It's all grace*, I think for the third time in about three minutes.

The best thing they do is gather Johanna up. We sit around the table; Johanna and I are in the center. Mari Anne offers up a prayer for the meal and asks for us to be guided by love and grace. She also asks for an extra measure of grace for me, and strength and patience for Johanna, and we start to eat. The meal is delicious, some sort of magical November soup that Lauren's created. The talk is fast. Everyone wants to know what we've been doing in the past ten days since my visit to the hospital. Everyone is solicitous but curious, and several times someone mentions, "Well, you look great. It's hard to believe you have anything wrong."

I suppose I look okay, but sometimes I wish the cancer had been more obvious. It seems unfair that there is no warning that something so insidious had invaded my body.

We finish dinner slowly because there is so much talking. "Where are the babies?" I ask Lauren, and she smiles.

"The twins are asleep, and the boys got to go to a movie with Dad."

Lauren has a great smile and gives the best hugs of anyone I know. She has now hugged me twice in passing this evening. Later in our friendship, she will tell me that she's trained herself to give strong hugs that last at least five seconds. She believes in the healing and loving quality of a good hug. She's right.

As dessert is passed around, Mari Anne announces that they have a surprise for me.

"Everyone pitched in and cooked soup for you, Bunny. We've loaded up Lauren's freezer with our soups and we're going to send them home with you. That way, when you or Johanna don't want to cook, you'll have soup to warm up."

I start to cry. I have been so overwhelmed with the news of my illness and the idea of Johanna having to come to live with me and the financial worries and about three million other concerns that I haven't even started to think about the cooking. Now I don't have to.

As the Bible study women load up bags with our containers of soup, I think of the months to come, when Johanna or I will be able to open one up and stick it in the microwave and get a little comfort. What I don't know is that, in addition to these soups, this group will feed us on the nights after each treatment by organizing meals for Wednesday and Thursday nights on chemo weeks. I will come home from chemo exhausted and washed out, and Johanna will have papers to write and homework to complete. There will be a ring of the doorbell, and someone we trust will show up with something hearty and delicious.

This is what care is all about. After another round of hugs and good wishes, Johanna and I make our way to the car, with Kristi and Lauren helping us with our bags of soup. After more hugs, we get into the car and head home.

"That was pretty amazing, Mom," Johanna says.

I look back at Lauren's wall. "Yes, it was, sweetie. It was amazing." I'm filled with emotion. And questions. What if I hadn't gotten cancer? What if these women hadn't had to band together to care for us? Is this as much for them as it is for me? Do they feel the grace as much as I do?

I don't know. I just know that, for tonight, I feel pretty full of love and grace. It's a good feeling. It's all grace.

When I get home, it is not difficult to know what to write: *Grateful for the Wine-Drinking Bible Study Group, for soup, for love, for Lauren, for grace.*

CHAPTER 14

Thanksgiving

∿➤

I have now been diagnosed for more than two weeks. I wonder if I can be more honest on CaringBridge. I write a lot about gratitude because it's what I know best right now. I'm not less pissed off at God and the cancer, but it feels like my job is to make everyone else feel good. Surely it will rub off on me at some point. I keep writing in the red notebook as well, although I have felt less optimistic than usual this past week. I have constant pain and a lot of fear and a general malaise about getting work done and moving forward. My insurance doesn't kick in until December 1. Some mornings, I think, *What's the point of doing anything until then?*

Regardless of how I feel, things are moving rapidly. I will have a houseful of company for Thanksgiving—Johanna, Zachary, and his pregnant wife, Lesley, are sleeping here. After my diagnosis, Zach called and asked if they could change their holiday plans. Getting cancer got my kids to change their original holiday plans. There's a benefit after all.

My nephew, Kene, his wife, Amy and their little girls, Courtney and Jimmy and two-year-old Ryver will all be staying in a Two Casitas house not far away. Some of my favorite people will be celebrating with me. I am surrounding myself with young couples and kids, thinking only about the food and how much beer and wine to buy and what we'll show Lesley on her first trip to Santa Fe.

I am trying not to think about the week following Thanksgiving, when the most serious medical procedures will begin. I'll have a PET scan and a port placement and then chemo, all within the first three days of December. I can't imagine what Christmas will be like.

Instead of thinking about it, I write something cheerful and full of gratitude, some of which I feel, some of which is manufactured.

CaringBridge Journal Entry — November 19, 2012

It's a beautiful Monday afternoon in Santa Fe, and I have my patio doors open, letting the sun and the clear autumn air in. My house is clean and winterized. All the leaves are raked. Thanks to Kent, Viola, Will, and Sarah for showing up yesterday to start on those chores and to Kent and Viola for staying until just a bit ago to finish. Not only did they work hard, we had great meals and lots of good conversation. While they cleaned up the yard, Sarah and I sat in the kitchen and talked about the holidays. Cancer patients like to hang together, I've learned.

Except for the cooking, I'm ready for Thanksgiving. My church friend Kelly is bringing over a pecan pie this evening. I don't know how to make one, and she offered. What a great gift.

On Thanksgiving Day, I will have my kids and best friends here. Our plan is food, football, napping, relaxation, and sitting around the newly assembled fire pit. With a fire burning, of course. We have much to be thankful for these days.

Despite all the gratitude I feel, I do have some dark moments. I work hard to not let them become dark days. On Friday afternoon, I had to go *back* to the Cancer Center for yet another CT scan, and the tech said, "Have you ever had one of these?"

I said, "Um, yeah, last Friday."

She gave me a puzzled look...and I had a flash of "What the hell am I doing here?"

I thought about being at the Cowgirl instead, or at the Plaza Cafe eating posole. Or soaking in a tub at Ten Thousand Waves. Or sitting at my mother's kitchen table visiting over coffee. Anything other than being shot up with yet another round of toxic chemicals that would make my organs glow in the dark. And I got angry—angry that I played by all the rules and didn't smoke and exercised and ate healthy foods, and I still got cancer. Some tears ran down the side of my face and into my ears as I lay on that table under the scan machine. And then I got over it. Because all the anger and tears in the universe will not make me well, nor will they make the cancer go away.

Tomorrow I go to the hospital for an EKG as part of the clinical study. I now know to take someone with me for those appointments, so that should be much better. Jennifer and her son, Josiah, will go with me for that one. What I know today is that I am not alone in any way.

Thanks for checking in. And Happy Thanksgiving!

After all the effort required to write that CaringBridge post, I don't write in the red notebook. Maybe tomorrow.

CHAPTER 15

Kakawa Chocolate and Being Brave

⌇⟶

Thanksgiving was all I wanted it to be. My house was full of young people who are my family and my friends. We cooked for hours and lingered over the meal and sat outside in the crisp November air that exists only in northern New Mexico. Someone in the neighborhood had piñon wood burning in their fireplace, and it made the world smell like a bowl of incense or a campfire high in the Sangre de Cristos. The kids drank a lot of beer, and each of the guys took a turn with Kene's guitar. Babies and toddlers played on the flagstone, and no one acted like I was an invalid. There were no tears.

Early on Friday morning, Kene and Amy came back from their Two Casitas condo toting croissants from Clafoutis. We had mimosas and relaxed in the living room while Lucy the Pug entertained Quinn, the baby girl.

There was an outing to the plaza where the City of Santa Fe had just lit the community Christmas tree. The balloon man made a puppy and a hat for my two-year-old great-niece, Kyle Jeanne, and we took a group photo of all the girls lined up on a bench. Just before the shutter snapped, Kyle turned and put her balloon hat on Lesley's head. We were all laughing. The photo doesn't show that anyone in the crowd was thinking about cancer.

Because we weren't.

But now the process begins. As of yesterday, I have health insurance and can begin all the procedures in earnest. Today is a PET scan. Tomorrow is port placement. Wednesday is chemo. This, even though the orientation nurse said they would have to wait two weeks after port placement to begin chemo. "The wound has to heal completely before we can pierce it with a needle," she said. And yet, Dr. L says that the minute the port is in, we need to begin chemo. There is some urgency to his statement.

A month ago, I was worrying about who would win the presidential election. Charlotte and I were talking about meeting at the Cowgirl to watch the election returns. I was getting on OkCupid and talking to Bob The Writer and thinking about how cool it would be if we had a meet and greet and liked each other enough to spend the holidays together.

Today I have a PET scan.

Johanna has made the transition and moved everything back to my house, but she has finals today. Jennifer will once again go with me to X-Ray Associates and sit in the waiting room with Josiah while they do my scan. Because the trial paid for it, I didn't have to wait for the insurance to kick in.

In the red notebook, I wrote, *Grateful for Jennifer and Josiah sitting in the waiting room, for T. J. calling every day, for Johanna moving back, for my parents praying over me every minute, for insurance.*

Last week, I had an interview with my clinical trial coordinator, and we talked about my demographics and medical history. I had no medical history of any kind to discuss, other than pregnancies and births. "I've never been sick," I said.

He replied, "Well, I have to be thorough. Twenty years down the road, this study will have proven exactly what we want it to prove."

For the study, I will receive a dose of Avastin with my 5FU every time I have chemo. There is talk of antibodies attaching to my cancer, or maybe my good cells. I should ask Jennifer. She takes the notes. In addition to the interview, I had an EKG scheduled at 1:00 at the hospital, and Jennifer asked to take me. I enthusiastically said yes, having learned that I'm better at these medical procedures if I know someone will be sitting in the waiting room when I'm done.

Because he's home-schooled, eight-year-old Josiah goes with us. He is an easy kid. He reminds me of Zachary at that age. The best thing about Josiah is that he's always laughing and smiling. Like his beautiful, patient mother, he's the perfect person to go with us to the hospital for a test.

Afterward, it seemed ridiculous to have taken them. The EKG turned out to be a nonevent. I was hooked up to a machine for thirty seconds. It took longer to put the sticky pads on my chest than to run the test. As we were climbing into the hospital security golf cart to be taken back to Jennifer's car on the lower-level parking lot, Josiah giggling about the ride, Jennifer announced that we were going to Kakawa Chocolate House for a treat.

I've never been to Kakawa Chocolate House, but I've heard about it. It's a specialty chocolate company whose "passion is authentic and historic drinking chocolates." We came in out of the cold like we owned the place. Josiah showed me to the case full of chocolates. He and I chose the dark chocolate with caramel and sea salt, and Jennifer and I sampled the hot chocolate elixirs. We settled on one each, and Josiah found us a table near a west window that looked across a parking lot to the Roundhouse.

And then I found my inspiration for the day. While she was paying for our treats, Jennifer told Josiah to count his carbs and check his levels. Josiah has juvenile diabetes. He checks his own levels, and just before having his chocolate of choice,

Jennifer gave him a quick injection of insulin, right there at our table, unobtrusively, with no one looking. There was not a moment of complaint, no little-boy sullenness, and no refusing his mother's requests. There was just Josiah's delight in his pyramid-shaped peanut butter chocolate treat and our deep discussion of how they created a mold that made the wedge look like it was bricked on the sides.

Josiah laughs, he smiles, he apparently enjoys every single moment of his existence. I've lived with a little boy, and I know there must be moments when he scrunches up his face and scowls at his mom when she tells him to do something like make his bed or take out the trash. But Josiah is a kid without complaint or fussiness, despite what has to be the continual headache of monitoring his sugar levels and a lifelong disease. And there is no complaint from Jennifer, either. They deal with his medical condition gracefully. That's what I want. That's who I want to be.

CHAPTER 16

No Stopping This Train

∿➤

I don't want to have a PET scan today. Last night, Stacy from the Wine-Drinking Bible Study group had a Christmas open house at her luxurious Palace Avenue home. It was a holiday event, with savory and sweet appetizers, wine, petit fours, and a home decorated to the nines. And cloth napkins, which, even at age fifty-one, still astound me. I've just never bothered to gather up any cloth napkins. Would I have if I had stayed married to that first Texas guy and created a true household instead of the movable feast that my life became because I was single? I don't know. I just know that I'm still easily impressed by people who have cloth napkins that have obviously been ironed. Crazy. Who has that much time?

For the twenty-four hours preceding the PET scan, I am not allowed to eat a single carb or anything with sugar, including alcohol. This is a hard thing to do with the Wine-Drinking Bible Study girls. They're in the holiday mood. I wonder if I'm bringing the party down.

The instructions say the PET scan will pick up on any energy in my body, especially carbs or sugar. This seems to be the theory on which people rest the notion that I can't eat any more sugar because cancer feeds on it. People tend to believe that sugar causes cancer. Some of my friends attack my eating habits as though I'm somehow responsible for my cancer. Is that possible?

I've already asked Dr. L about this theory. He shakes his head, saying, "As though cancer discriminates and only chooses people who have eaten sugar. Cancer does not discriminate." He says everyone has a theory and that it's their way of making sense of the horrors of the disease. I think horror is a word he could have left out of the conversation, but he's right. It is a horror.

At Stacy's, I had something wrapped in bacon that had absolutely no carbs. I looked longingly at everything else, especially the homemade fudge. I love fudge.

Stacy's mother was visiting with a group of women from the Dallas area. They all very sweetly put their hands on my arm and said they had heard about me and were praying for me. I thanked them, turned away, and had to go into the bathroom for a minute. I am alternately touched and repelled by people's concern for me. I don't know why. Why can't I just be gracious and say, "That's so kind. I appreciate it," and let it go at that? Why do I have to get a bit bristly when people are kind? Is it because this is so new?

Maybe I just have too much on my mind. My head is full of the events of this week. I am petrified about the port placement and then the chemo following so quickly the day after. Will I be bald this time next week? Will I forget I have the line into my port for infusion and roll over in the night and disconnect myself, spilling chemo all over the bed sheets?

Regardless of how weirded out I am about my life and the cancer, I am thankful for these women. At the end of the evening, when we've visited and talked about prayer in general, I am the first person on the prayer request list. Mari Anne always looks at me with those blue eyes and says, "What exactly do you want us to pray for?" before she asks anyone else. I worry that people leave stuff off the prayer list because they think my issues are too big. One of the women is single and facing a layoff, and my heart aches for her. She's understandably scared and emotional, but instead of sharing, she looks at me and says, "But it's not that big a deal." I hate this role. I hate being the person whose needs outweigh everyone else's.

At the same time, I'm overwhelmed with the support I get from these women. They've already organized the food posse, as promised, and one of them will bring us an evening meal for the day of chemo and for each subsequent day I'm on the pump. They're prepared for this coming Wednesday, Thursday, and Friday, even if I'm not.

Mari Anne prays such eloquent prayers. It feels like God is in the room, sitting across the coffee table from us, putting His hand on my head while she asks for grace and courage and no pain, and finally for healing. I could sit right here in this circle of women forever.

I go out into the December night to find my car and look up at the sky. The stars are bright, and because there is so little light pollution, this feels almost like the nights when I'd go out on my deck at the lake in Logan and gaze at the sky. It is the beginning of the Christmas season, and tomorrow I start doing stuff that has nothing to do with holiday cheer. Thank goodness for the prayers. I'm going to need them.

For the Wine-Drinking Bible Study Group, for my clients who keep sending me work, for my dad calling today, for getting started, for Ambien.

We are moving forward. There is no stopping this train now.

CHAPTER 17

Larry McMurtry and the Day Before Chemo

∿➤

I just finished reading *Leaving Cheyenne* by Larry McMurtry again. I'm sitting on my patio on an unseasonably warm December afternoon, tears running down my face. It's not as if I didn't already know that Gid would die on the way to the hospital in Wichita Falls, that Johnny would turn around at the red light and know for sure that his friend of sixty-two years had stopped breathing in the backseat. I knew when they started working on that windmill, replacing the sucker rod and the old pipe, that Gid would fall off the ladder, get a blood clot, and die, thinking he'd been thrown by a horse up on the plains of the Panhandle, thinking he was twenty-two instead of sixty-six. I know all that. It's not as if I haven't read the book at least forty times. The cover is torn and coming apart from so many late nights in a steamy tub with me. The first time I read it, Zach was a baby. Now he's about to have a baby of his own.

It's not really Gid's dying that has me in tears. It's more that I want to be Molly, living in the country, gathering the eggs and loving cowboys, getting in the storm cellar when there's a tornado threatening in the distance, cleaning out the hayloft and finding relics from my childhood. I want to bake cornbread and feed it to my boys on the porch with buttermilk for dessert. I want to go fishing at the dirt tank and fry the catfish over an open fire.

What I want most of all is to not have to go to chemo tomorrow.

I think, *I have no business living in the city like this. I am a child of the country.* I grew up on a farm in rural Quay County. For all my love of having the Cowgirl and pizza delivery and Double Take Consignment down the road, I still long for my own cowboy or two, a couple of good old boys to fight over my affection. I know my Santa Fe girlfriends would argue that I'm not being feminist enough, that I'm selling myself short having these thoughts. But what I want this evening is the comfort of knowing that some man is loving me in the most old-fashioned way.

I also think, *I have no business having cancer or a new scar from my port placement.* The port was put in today and it hurts, the tumor continues to be painful, and I am about to become a walking science experiment. I don't want to be paying this exorbitant rent. I want to be in my house on a farm or ranch somewhere going through seed catalogs, planning next year's garden.

Maybe McMurtry and missing a life with cowboys are only excuses for the tears, and the chemo is the real reason. I'm not ready, except that I am. I don't want those off-the-charts chemicals in my body, yet I do. I want my tumors to start shrinking immediately, and I want to be well tomorrow. Dr. L says if the chemo works, the relentless stitch in my side will go away and I'll feel better almost instantly. He also says the chemo might (most certainly will) make me feel worse elsewhere.

I want to be well the moment the chemo enters my bloodstream. But that's not what will happen. Instead, they'll poke a large needle in my just-installed catheter port, and I'll sit in the chemo suite with Johanna. I'll get a dose of steroids and anti-nausea medicine and the Avastin that is the study drug and then three bags of chemo medicine.

The orientation nurse told me chemo treatments take at least five hours the first time. Johanna has packed a snack and drink bag, with ginger snaps for nausea, a banana for potassium, some beef jerky for protein, and coconut water for added nutrition. We'll take our computers and books, and she's taking her knitting.

I don't want to go. I want to stay at home on the farm with Gid or Johnny or whatever other man is out there that I shouldn't have turned down all those years ago when we were all choosing mates. Right now, I don't know why I was so stubborn or picky. It would be so nice to have a man in my life to carry some of this worry around. Where is the sweet cowboy in my life?

I don't write anything in the red notebook. I should probably write that I'm grateful that I finally stopped crying, but I can't even say that with any conviction. I cry into the night and hope for the best.

CHAPTER 18

Chemo Number One and Pot in a Teacup

∿➤

I did it. I had my first chemo treatment. Before we left the house, I wrote, *Grateful to get started. That's all.*

Johanna and I showed up for an appointment with Dr. L at 8:30 a.m. He looked at my port scar and said, "Well, that looks pretty good for just having been placed yesterday."

It's a lie. It is an angry red wound, but my skin is glued together and covered with some sort of transparent dressing that the radiologist said will keep it sealed and shielded from infection. There are no stitches, just a dark red line under the plastic. As Sarah said, it is uglier than sin.

The port placement was horrid. There is no other word. I was frightened and sweaty, and then I was out like a light, for maybe twenty minutes. Afterward, there was an *appliance* under my skin, just above my collarbone on the right side. It is painful and awkward, a bump where there wasn't one before. I held an ice pack on it, twenty minutes on, twenty minutes off, all day long. It had to be ready for chemo today.

The radiological oncologist said before the placement, "So you start chemo in a couple of weeks?"

"Um, no, tomorrow," I said, and he tried to hide his surprise. Usually, a port placement has to heal for a couple of weeks before they go in with a needle and chemicals. Because of my "now I finally have insurance" status, there is a rush to get everything done in a hurry. The tumors are growing daily. Fucking cancer. My Southern Baptist Grandma would roll over in her grave to hear me talk like this, and probably God, wherever He might be hiding, isn't too thrilled with it, either, but my prayer is that I can just be my totally pissed-off self today without retribution.

After he admired what he called my "good-looking port placement," Dr. L let us know that my CEA has shot up from an original 67 to 82. Which means that we probably caught this just in time. I'll learn later that some colon cancer patients never have an elevated CEA. Right now, I'm not excited about those numbers, but eventually I'll be relieved that I have this indicator of how I'm doing and whether the chemo is working.

I ask him again how many chemo treatments I'll have to have and how long this will take. He very patiently says that we shouldn't get in a hurry and that it will probably be around six. For some reason, Johanna and I hear this as six weeks. That is not exciting, but doable. We'll learn later that we heard him incorrectly. Six treatments equal twelve weeks. I'll have a treatment every two weeks and be hooked up for forty-eight hours to a pump, with a disconnect on Fridays.

What I hear him saying, without saying it aloud, is that he doesn't really have a clue how this will go and we shouldn't get ahead of ourselves.

We go to the chemo suite. I write a CaringBridge post that sugarcoats what is one of the worst experiences of my life. Everyone at home wants details. Before we left home this morning, I talked to my parents, to my sister, to one of my brothers, to my friend, Angie, and to my niece, Amy. I need to send out some news, and it needs to be good. This is what I write:

I woke up with John Fogerty's "Center Field" running through my brain. It was my mantra for the day. Put me in, coach.

I was ready to go, ready to get in the game, ready to get this first round of chemo behind me. Johanna and I got to the cancer center at 8:00 a.m. and had lab work, doctor visit, and then chemo. We're still here at 2:30, but the word from Mary Kay, our incredibly capable and friendly nurse, is that we're less than a half hour from going home.

The chemo has been uneventful, mostly. The chemo suite is a beautiful place with a view of the Sangre de Cristos. Volunteers circulate with snacks and bring us juice and coffee and water and blankets and anything we might want in the world, except margaritas. I'm going to have to speak to the administration about that lapse.

Jennifer came at noon and gave Johanna a break. Josiah sat out in the waiting room in my line of vision and gave me a wave every once in a while. Will's girlfriend and my cancer mentor, Sarah, happened to be here for her monthly treatment, so we visited back and forth. The other patients are friendly, relaxed, and in varied stages of health, but still, nobody is badly behaved or seeming very unhappy.

All in all, it has been mostly a social event with an IV attached. And you all know how I love myself a social event.

I will go home with a pump attached to my port that will pump chemo for the next forty-six hours. I'll come back on Friday for that to be removed. In between all that, we get to have dinner with Jennifer and Drew and the boys tonight, maybe dinner tomorrow at Kristi Hartley Hunt's, and a couple of days to relax at home.

As my mom said this morning on the phone after she and Dad prayed over me, "It's all an adventure." I've now had port placement and a PET scan, and this is the last procedure of the week. It's all going to be fine. Thanks for checking in.

I read that post a day later, with eighteen hours still left on the pump, and I can't believe how optimistic I was. Right after I typed that falsely cheerful chemo status, the irenotecan took hold and knocked me on my ass. I had a severe hot flash, the first of my life. I was sweating, wanting to tear my clothes off. My nose started running, with snot dripping down onto my lips. My eyes were itchy and wet. Johanna handed me a box of Kleenex and went for Mary Kay.

"This happens sometimes," she said, and offered me a shot of something to lessen the symptoms.

"Please, anything. This is making me crazy," I said. I wanted to cry, but I couldn't get my head straight enough to even know what was happening. I was burning up from the inside.

She stuck a hypodermic needle into my IV, and I immediately started to feel some relief. There was also some dizziness, but she assured me it would go away. It was a side effect of the injection. My head was swimming, but I no longer felt like I was on fire.

As the last of the chemo dripped through the line, she brought me my black pouch with the kangaroo symbol on the outside. It looks like an extra-long fanny pack and has straps that go around my waist or my shoulder, my choice. Just as Sarah did earlier in the day, Mary Kay suggested I wear it around my waist since this is new to me. She showed me the infusion pump that is placed in the pack. It's loaded with Folfiri/5FU, the chemo cocktail I ended up with in the study. It dispenses a dose every ninety seconds over a period of forty-six hours.

Johanna had to help me to the car. I was so dizzy from the injection Mary Kay had given me that I couldn't walk on my own. I got into my car hot and dizzy, with my nose no longer running but itchy. The bandages over my port were itchy as well, and the tube running from the port to the infuser made me nervous. I was afraid I'd catch the line on something and rip my chest open. My mind was a jumble of discomfort and heat and instructions and dizziness.

It was clear that dinner with Jennifer and her family wasn't going to happen. I wasn't able to walk, much less make conversation, especially with her three young boys looking on. I never wanted to eat again anyway, so food wasn't an issue. I kept waiting for the steroids to kick in, to make me feel strong and hungry. That's what Dr. L had promised. All I felt was whiny, exhausted, dizzy, and mostly fragile, which was new and hateful for me.

Johanna got me home, and I collapsed on the red couch. I had a blinding headache. After an hour or two, she phoned the nurse on call and asked what we could do for the headache. Advil was the suggestion, so I took four. No relief. I drank water, even though my mouth tasted like a roll of dirty nickels. I tried to think of something I wanted to eat.

Johanna looked through the soups the Bible study girls gave us to keep in the freezer. "Butternut squash?" she asked. "Chicken and dumplings?"

"You choose," I told her. I had no desire to eat anything.

I thought again about how I hated this for her, but how I couldn't do it without her. I was flat on my back with a raging headache, a tube coming out of my chest, no appetite, and my nose was running again. I also had vertigo. Resting my head against a surface made the room swing in circles. I reached out to hold onto the coffee table, and the dizziness subsided, but not much.

From this treatment forward, I'd learn to refuse the second med that stopped the hot flash and the runny nose. I'd know that I could tolerate those first symptoms better than the dizziness. My nose would run, and after the second treatment, it would start to bleed without warning. My gums would bleed as well, and my contacts would be so uncomfortable that I'd have to stop wearing them for long periods of time.

But for now, I just had to get through the first evening of the first day of chemo.

I tried to remember Martin's prayer about the blinders. I tried to think of five things to be grateful for, but all I had was *Johanna, Johanna, Johanna.*

My cell phone rang every few minutes. Johanna had silenced hers, but I saw that she was checking it often. Zachary, my parents, my siblings, my friends. Everyone wanted a report from the first day of chemo. Johanna handled all the calls while I sat very still on the couch and tried to stop the room from spinning and the headache from splitting my head wide open.

We learned that the only cure for my headache was pot. Not Advil, not pain meds. A week later, I'd go to my favorite restaurant/bar and ask my favorite waiter in the most round-about way what one should do if one was getting a certain kind of treatment and one needed some herbal relief, but one was new in town and didn't really know where to find that sort of thing.

He'd look at me and say, "You're not talking about you, are you?" I'd say yes, and he'd hang his head for a minute and tell me to go back and sit at my table. In less than five minutes, he'd stop by the table and set a Styrofoam cup with a lid and a tea bag on top of the lid in front of me.

"Drink your tea and stay well, Bunny. Stay well."

Inside the cup would be three fat buds of pot. After everything was said and done, marijuana would be the only thing that made my post-chemo evenings tolerable.

The Cancer Center tells me they won't give me a prescription for medical marijuana, but they will give me the names of a dispensary and a doctor from whom I can get one. It seems like too much of a hassle, which is how everything seems right now. I'll learn where I can scavenge some weed now and then. I won't smoke it, but I'll eat it in brownies. It will be the only thing that works for my headaches. Not hydrocodone, not oxycontin, not any of my other meds. I will want to write about it in my little red notebook but won't. It's silly that it's illegal, but it is.

I hate being on the pump. I am tethered to a plastic line that goes from my port to my fanny pack of chemo. My anxiety about the line adds to my already overwhelming physical discomfort. I am tentative about moving around. I certainly don't want to go out of the house until I'm disconnected. The day after my first treatment, I spend most of the morning soaking in the tub, careful to keep my shoulders and my angry red port incision out of the water. I'm still too new at this to try a shower, although I know the line is long enough that I could leave the infusion pump on the counter and step into the stall. After the bath, I dress. I have to figure out how to weave the line through or under my clothing so I can then belt it to my hip.

At night in bed, I put the pump on my bedside table and worry about rolling over onto my port and the line. There's no chance of that though, because the one time I start to do it, the needle poking into my port shifts and hurts like a son of a bitch. I think back to last week, when I was wishing I had a man in my bed. Now I know what a bad idea that was; the whirring of the pump every ninety seconds is enough to drive me crazy. It's not loud, just insistent. And the dressing and the bulkiness of the port are anything but sexy. Just as I suspected, I am never going to have sex again.

And I'm going to go crazy before this pump comes out.

And then of course, I could die.

But don't think about that. Not going to happen.

A digital reading tells me how much F5U has been infused and how much is left in the pump. I started with 110 ml, and in the middle of the night, it says I now have 67. I calculate I'm infusing at a rate of 2.2 ml per hour, so I now have less than thirty-three hours to go. Or something like that. I still have a headache, but I've taken about a dozen Advil and a couple hydrocodone, and its less painful than before.

What I didn't gamble on was the steroids keeping me awake. Like that cocaine we all tried in the '80s, this is an awake that has my body exhausted but my mind racing and my eyes wide open. There is no sleep to be had.

At 3:00 a.m., I finally take another Ambien. It's not like I have to be anywhere tomorrow. Hell, I'm a cancer patient. I can sleep in until noon if I want. While the pump whirs and my heart races, I try to meditate or pray myself to sleep. I hear my dad saying, "If I were any better, I'd have to be two people." He's right. I have the best medical care possible, I have Johanna, and I have him and my mom. I have hundreds of people cheering on the sidelines for my recovery.

This is treatment number one. Only eleven to go, according to the sign Johanna put on my desk today. She also left a note on my mirror in the bathroom that says, "Whatever happens, we are in this *together*."

Boy, do I love that girl. We may make it after all. If I can just get some sleep first.

I take out the red notebook. *Zachary, Johanna, Mom, Dad, Ambien. First day done.*

CHAPTER 19

2% Chance of Survival

⤳

Here are the rules I've learned so far about cancer and chemo: Rest. Take lots of iron. Then take magnesium to combat the constipation from the iron. Don't be in large crowds because my white count will be low from the chemo. Don't take Vitamin C because it's an antioxidant, and chemo is an oxidant. Don't take aspirin or Tylenol, *ever*, or I can't have chemo for two weeks. Don't get on the internet. Don't get on the internet. Don't get on the internet. That was Dr. L's strongest advice. Sarah's, too.

Last night, on the second day after chemo, while my fanny pack whirred every ninety seconds, I sat at my computer and read my emails. No cancer research this time. I checked out Facebook, where I have a cheering section of thousands. The love and encouragement is stunning. Sometimes it makes me cry to read the comments on Johanna's updates about how I'm doing.

Someone from my hometown sent me a Facebook message with a link to an alternative treatment center in Phoenix specializing in stage IV cancers. She suggested that I go there for another opinion. This came from someone that I haven't spoken to in years. We don't run in the same circles. She's just a person who went to high school with my brother.

Of course I click on the link. I'm crazy that way.

The first thing I see is an infographic dominating the corner of the center's colon cancer info page. It says my five-year chance of survival with stage IV cancer is 2%.

2% That's a very small number. Scary. If you don't watch out, that number will make you cry. That means that this place thinks 98% of the patients in my shoes will be dead in less than five years.

I turn off my computer.

Throughout the night, I keep waking with "2%" in my brain. I'm already having a hard time sleeping because of the steroids. Every time I open my eyes, I think of my first grand-child, a baby boy, coming in March. I dream of taking him hiking in the Pecos, of going to the Museum of International Folk Art to show him the Girard Collection and the dioramas his dad and Aunt Johanna loved as children. I picture a wintry day on the plaza with him, the balloon guy shaping a puppy and a hat from long, skinny balloons. I see him on the beach at Ute Lake, playing in the sand.

Then I remember "2%" and think how the odds had not always seemed that much in my favor for some things. Like big-money jobs. Or happy marriages. Or great boyfriends who take care of stuff so I don't have to do every damn thing. Maybe now it's my turn for the odds to swing in my favor.

But 2%?

One tiny bit of advice to anyone out there who knows someone with cancer: Don't send these links. It's an ugly, inconsiderate thing to do, even when you want to be helpful. If you're sending a link, read every single word of that website or article before you send it out, and make damn sure it's only encouraging, that it says we'll all get well, and chemo won't be hard, and everything is going to work out perfectly. Because right now, at this stage of the game, I don't need to read anything that says otherwise.

2%. Holy shit. That will keep you awake at night, despite two Ambiens.

In the morning, I get up and send an email to the Bible study women and tell them exactly what happened. I ask them to pray for me to forget that number because I cannot fight this fight when all I see is Baby Nolan doing all those things without me.

I get out the red notebook. *Baby coming, Ambien, Bible study women.* It's all I can think of right now.

CHAPTER 20

Happy Birthday to Me

∿➤

My birthday is December 8, which will be exactly thirty days after I went to the ER with a stitch in my side. When I didn't have cancer, Courtney, Amy, and Angie, my girlfriends from Logan, made a plan to spend my birthday weekend with me so we could go dancing at the Cowgirl and have margaritas at Del Charro and a spa treatment or two. It was a vague plan that sounded like a perfect birthday weekend for a fifty-two-year-old and her friends.

Instead, my birthday is three days after my first chemo treatment, the day the orientation nurse said would be my worst day. "You'll be exhausted," she said. "The steroids will have worn off, and your body will feel like you've deflated."

I'm pretty sure dancing at the Cowgirl and drinks at Del Charro aren't on the list of smart things to do, given the circumstances.

I talk to T. J. every single day, more than anyone else. He extracted a promise that I'd always answer when he called. "Robin and I want to hear from you and know how you're doing," he said with a catch in his voice. So I call him every day, sometimes twice. If I don't call him, he calls me. Because he is not only my cousin but my business partner, we frequently start with a conversation about real estate. It gives us a way to pretend that the calls are necessary for the business rather than because I need to unload on someone who is not Johanna or Zach or my parents.

On Thursday when I'm on the pump, he asks me what I'm doing for my birthday. "Resting, I guess," I say. "Maybe Johanna will go to storage and get the Christmas tree." I'm already tired thinking about Christmas. The chemo has given me a headache that won't go away.

"What if Taylor and Robin and I come up and help with the Christmas tree? And take you to dinner for your birthday?" T. J. says, and I know he wants to see me and reassure himself that I'm still standing. "Can you get us one of Wendy's Two Casitas houses?"

I am relieved. I am so exhausted with trying to hold the idea of Christmas in my head, with the lists of events and gifts to be purchased (*ordered*, I think, because I never want to leave this couch) and decorations to be hauled out and put up. Anyone in this situation might forgo decorating, but even if I'm sick, I'm stubborn. This is my first Christmas in Santa Fe, Johanna is here, and we will, dammit, celebrate.

But T. J. and Robin know me better than anyone else right now. Their offering to do this is the answer I didn't know I wanted. Adding Taylor to the mix is even better. He and Johanna are the same age, cousins who graduated from high school together, and he will make her feel more normal in this week of weirdness.

I call Wendy at Two Casitas and ask for a house. She is, as always, helpful without being intrusive. I have learned the difference. When I say what I need, some people say, "Great, let me handle that for you." Others want to get in the middle of what's happening, asking for details. If I have any surprise reaction to cancer and its attendant conditions, it is that I am sick to death of talking, talking, talking about the cancer and about myself. I've always liked to talk. However, now I hate talking about cancer.

Wendy and I have an understanding. I write blogs about Santa Fe and her properties, and in return, she gives me a weekend each month in the homes she manages. It's a barter system that helped me decide to move here. Back in January when I was wallowing in self-pity because I had just been ugly-dumped by Last Boyfriend, she approached me with this proposal. It's a gift to both of us. My blogs help her business and online presence; her weekend stays helped me fall in love all over again with this city.

And now Wendy doesn't ask me to talk about how I'm doing. She simply says, "I've got a great house they can stay in. I hope you're having an okay day." Her kindness makes me cry. I thank her and say that yeah, the day is not terrible, and she gives me the address and the code to get in the door.

Johanna drives me to the "casita" Wendy gives us for the weekend. It's not a casita, however. It's a luxurious house on a hill just above Canyon Road, with three kiva fireplaces and views of both the Jemez Mountains and the Sangre de Cristos. It's the most beautiful Two Casitas property I've ever seen. I want to build a fire in one of the fireplaces and stay here for the night. Instead, I leave the porch light on and turn up the heat. I'm grateful to Wendy for taking such good care of us. My trade of writing content for her website in exchange for homes to stay in has turned out to be one of the best business deals I've ever made.

Then it is Saturday morning and my birthday. T. J., Robin, and Taylor arrived in Santa Fe after midnight last night and texted us at 10:00 this morning. "Breakfast at Tecolote's?" is what the text says, and I am happy to hear from them. I woke up feeling almost spry, compared to the past three days. I'm off the pump. I didn't spill chemo on myself. I didn't throw up once. I still have my hair. It is early days, but I feel close to human.

"Yes!" I text back. They come by and pick us up in their bright red Dodge pickup and life immediately improves. Here we are, with our best pals who are also family. The sun is shining, and Johanna and I are getting out of the house and away from just each other. We need this respite from our daily life. It feels joyful.

After Huevos Zacatecas that I mostly don't eat, pushing the plantains around the plate in an attempt to make it look as if I'm wolfing it down, we go to the storage unit for the decorations. Every trip down Cerrillos Road with T. J. is an adventure. He is like me, always on the lookout for something new and interesting and fun. We should have been siblings instead of cousins.

Back when I had determined that I was going to starve myself financially if I stayed in Logan and tried to continue running my coffee shop, I called T. J. "I have an idea," I told him and proceeded to relay my plans for starting a new real estate business involving him, Robin, my brother, Kent, and his wife, Viola. I knew from experience that T. J. made things happen, that his energy and common sense and street smarts, but mostly his ambition, would serve a business well. He would not allow us to fail. I thought we could combine that with Kent's knowledge of the area and make something successful for all of us.

Even when Kent and Viola opted out of the partnership after a few years, I stayed, and T. J. and Robin and I have continued to be business partners in the best sense of the word. We all have separate strengths that help the business thrive. And in all those days spent in the office together, our old friendships have gotten bigger and better and closer.

Watching T. J., Taylor, and Johanna load the boxes of decorations into the back of the pickup makes me feel comforted and happy in a way that I haven't been in a couple of weeks. Now things will be taken care of, and I won't have to think about Johanna being shortchanged out of Christmas this year.

It is threatening snow in that crazy Santa Fe way. The sun is shining, but the air is crisp, and the Sangre de Cristos are obscured by clouds. We spend the day putting up the 1960s aluminum tree I ordered from eBay years ago, hanging garland from the white picket fence outside and wrapping holly around the portal posts. Or rather, they work, and I watch. Sometimes I lie down on the red couch with a book and think about how good my life is, mostly. Today is my birthday. I am fifty-two years old. I have stage IV cancer. This is freaking crazy.

The snow starts just as the sun is going down. We are going to go to La Casa Sena for dinner to celebrate my birthday. I know exactly what I will order — the flank steak with the side dish, a roasted green chile stuffed with mashed potatoes and covered with cheese. I swear I will eat all of it. It is one of my favorite dishes in the world, and I need to eat as much red meat as possible. I take an iron pill every day, but my hemoglobin remains precariously low. I swear I will eat every bite. It is my birthday.

After dinner, I know we'll walk to the plaza, where every tree is hung with different colored lights. I love Christmas in Santa Fe. This is one of the reasons I moved here — it is nothing short of magical. Too bad I have cancer for my first Christmas here, but I still get to be here for the holiday. I still get to walk the plaza under those lit trees. And my best friends and family will do it with me.

I guess I've dozed off on the red couch because the side door opens and cold air rushes in. T. J. comes in and gets me off the couch. "Come see what we've done," he says. I stumble into my coat and boots and follow him outside.

It is dusk, that very first dark of early evening. Snow is falling softly as he leads me out to the street in front of my adobe house. Taylor, Robin, and Johanna stand in the street waiting on me, and I turn to look at the house. They have strung lights along the lip of the roof of the portal and wound them around the support columns. They've hung them on the picket fence, and there's garland in great strands around the fence as well. There is a green wreath with a bow on the front door. I can see Johanna's little Christmas tree lit up through a window in her bedroom.

I begin to cry, and Robin is crying with me. This is exactly the birthday I wanted and needed right this minute. My house is beautiful, Christmas is going to get here, and I'm going to be okay.

Before I go to sleep that night, I fill the red notebook with more than five things: *T J. and Rob, Johanna and Taylor, Christmas coming, my old aluminum tree, the snow, dinner at La Casa Sena, the plaza, being off the pump, feeling good.*

Chapter 21

Small Towns and Big Love

~~→

We're having a meeting tonight to plan a benefit for you," T. J. says the next week at the end of our daily conversation, during which we talked about my fatigue and his trying to sell one of the ranches we have listed and the basketball season starting up this month at Logan High. I want the ranch to sell, and I want to be able to go home for basketball games.

I love going to high school basketball games. Dr. L says to avoid large crowds because of my potentially damaged white blood cell count, so I guess the basketball will have to wait.

"A benefit?" I ask.

"Yeah. Folks around here sure do seem to want to do something for you. You're kind of a rock star or something," he says with a laugh and a sigh.

It's true. Johanna says I'm like a rock star without the talent or the cash. People want to talk to me, see me, and be in my presence. I get it for the ones who have always known and loved me. Not so much for everyone else. But it's nice that the people in Logan, population 1,100, with an economy that's none too strong, want to go to the trouble of raising money for my fight with cancer.

We discuss dates, and I say that if it's possible, I want it to be sooner rather than later. According to everyone at the Cancer Center, the first two treatments won't be physically difficult, other than the runny nose, dizziness, and fatigue. Then, evidently, the chemo will build up in my system, and each subsequent treatment will make me feel worse. I'm having my second treatment on December 19, the Wednesday before Christmas.

"Obviously, we can't do it before Christmas, but how about right after?" he says.

"I guess that will work, and I guess I'll actually have to be there?" I ask, filled with dread at the idea of being the center of everyone's attention just because I have cancer. I used to love a crowd. I was a social butterfly in the worst sense of the word. I don't even know if I was likable, but I loved to get in a crowd and talk to everyone at once. Now I dread having to see people who will fawn over me and treat me like a sick person.

I'm reminded how the cancer diagnosis has changed me. I used to be more fun. I used to be the person everyone wanted to join them for a party or a weekend or a day on the lake. I talked, I laughed, I danced. I lived my life with abandon and reminded myself every day how every moment was enormous, and it was all we had, thanks to Natalie Goldberg. I talked about death every day with my kids or friends because I had heard that was a Zen practice, and it made sense to me that talking about death was a way to live a bigger life. I believed and repeated to myself every day that if my life were any better, I'd have to be two people. I knew my dad had it right.

Now I seem to have folded in on myself. It's like all that theory that I espoused in my life before cancer now needs to be put into practice, and I'm too paralyzed by reality to do it. I almost feel like a different person. The only thing that keeps me grounded in that old way of thinking is the gratitude notebook, and most days, I write those lines only because of habit.

"Yes, goofball, you have to be at your own benefit," T. J. tells me.

And so the planning begins. I hear from Courtney and Angie that the first planning meeting in the Logan High School Library goes relatively well, until my mom, dad, sister, and brothers show up and everyone dissolves into tears. I'm relieved that I'm not living in Logan these days, although it would be lovely to be around my family. The continual emotion could be gut-wrenching.

Don't get me wrong. I appreciate everyone's good wishes and care and kindness. I am just so overwhelmed by my own emotions that I'm incapable of handling anyone else's. And as Johanna says, we'd like to believe that cancer is not the only thing happening in our lives. In Santa Fe, we can go out for dinner, to the movies, or to a gallery opening, and not a soul in the room knows about the cancer. I look just like everyone else, although sometimes I'm carrying an ugly whirring fanny pack. This wouldn't work in Logan.

At the benefit meeting, there was talk of how to do it. T. J. reports later that everyone said, "Bunny should be here. She's the one who always plans these things."

It's true. I'm good at putting together an event, especially a benefit. When Logan's beloved school secretary had a stroke and was in a nursing home needing exploratory surgery that insurance wouldn't cover, my mom and I and a crew of locals put together an auction and dinner that raised more than $21,000 for her family in one day. When a third-grader from our church was in ICU for several days, we created a Death by Chocolate evening that netted more than $5,000 in about two hours.

But it wasn't my being involved that made these things happen. It was the generosity of my hometown, a place where the median income is probably hovering around $35,000 annually, but where they're all willing to throw a hundred-dollar bill into a donation jar, write a check, or bake a pie for a pie auction. Logan takes care of its own.

The Annex Bar and Grill, owned by my generous cousins, offers to provide all the food for a green chile enchilada supper at the school cafeteria. I don't have to do anything other than provide a photo for the posters and okay the raffle of several guns. I personally hate guns other than for hunting, but I am a Quay County girl and I know the items that will bring in the most cash are guns.

T. J. is put in charge. He makes things happen, and he and Robin are supreme organizers. We've both been on the board of the Chamber of Commerce for years now. He can hold hundreds of details in his head.

Shelley will arrange for use of the school and the logistics. She and I have been friends since second grade. She stood up with me at my first wedding out at Ute Lake. She'll gather her family, who is like my own, and they'll all set up, serve, and man the silent auction and the raffles. I'm hearing about these plans without concerning myself with them. I trust my friends to handle the details. For once, it's not my job.

I'm instead thinking about my next chemo treatment and my out-of-pocket medical expenses and my deductible, both of which have to be met before the end of the year. Five thousand dollars in out-of-pocket expenses, a deductible of $1,000. Today a statement came that says each chemo treatment is costing my insurance company about $11,000 every four weeks. I'll have to pay $1,000 for the deductible immediately and then pay $1,100 for my 20 percent, and then I'll have another treatment on the 19th. Is that $3,100 before the end of the year? I'm also getting bills from my uninsured hospital stay. Numbers spin through my head. I see my little nest egg of Logan home equity I had socked away for a Santa Fe property dwindling daily.

I now owe Christus St. Vincent more than $18,000, and that doesn't include the ER doctor or the tacky gastroenterologist who said my cancer "might" be treatable.

Maybe a benefit isn't a bad idea. I ask that they have a dance, just so I can do some serious dancing before I'm completely laid out by the chemo. They agree. When you're a cancer rock star, people try to accommodate your wishes.

In the red notebook, which is filling up quickly because I know I have to put a positive spin on my situation, I write, *Nest egg, benefit, Jeanne taking us to lunch again, Johanna's finals being over, Mom and Dad.* I have to stop worrying about money. I absolutely have to.

CHAPTER 22

Dread, Positive Thoughts, Dread

∿➤

For the second treatment, Johanna and I are all business. She had our bag packed the night before with snacks, water bottles, and my fanny pack for the infusion machine. I had blood tests on Monday, which is the way it will go from now on. I got the all-clear to proceed with today's treatment.

This is so Johanna. She is organized and has been her entire life. When she was starting kindergarten, she found comfort in having her backpack ready and waiting by the front door and her clothes laid out every night. She was living with two people who were flying by the seats of their pants. Zachary sometimes slept in the clothes he wore the day before. I rushed around every morning, throwing something in the dryer to get the wrinkles out, searching for my keys and my purse.

Meanwhile, little Johanna stood patiently waiting for us to get our acts together and get in the car to drive to school. It was adorable, most of the time. Now it's a relief. I don't have to think about anything. She was born for this role.

Here's how our schedule works now. Every other week, we will have blood tests at the Cancer Center on Monday, followed by an oncologist consult early Wednesday morning, in which Dr. L and my trial coordinator will look at my blood test results to see how I'm doing. After the consult, Johanna and I will go upstairs to the chemo suite for a day of treatment. After chemo, I'll be hooked to the pump, which I will wear in that goofy fanny pack, for about forty-two hours. Disconnect on Friday. This will all become second nature in the coming months, but I will never wake on a Wednesday chemo morning thinking happy thoughts. My only positive thought is that Johanna will have everything ready.

The big deal is the blood work. Because my CEA was 69 in the hospital and climbed to 82 right before my first treatment, Dr. L is ordering that we check it every two weeks. Normal CEA hovers at or below five. This test will be one of the ways we know the chemo is working. I want this chemo to work. I don't want to be doing all this for nothing. The port alone is so ugly that this absolutely must be working.

This morning, we put our bags and our laptops in the backseat of the car and head to the cancer center. My port incision hurts, but Jennifer created a small gray flannel pillow decorated with bits of bright fabric. I wear that over the incision when I buckle my seatbelt across it. I am so thankful for Jennifer's presence in our crazy lives right now. She is the backup for whatever Johanna needs.

I'm also grateful for the beautiful place where I go for doctor visits and chemo treatments. At least I don't have to face ugly surroundings. I think about the view of the Sangre de Cristos from the chemo suite chairs. I think of Mary Pat, the nice nurse I had last time. Maybe I'll have her again. It's the luck of the draw, but I want a nurse I can trust. There's one who is already giving me bad vibes. But I can't think about her. I have decided that I will view this cancer adventure only with as many positive thoughts as I can summon in the middle of my dread. Being frightened of a chemo suite nurse who I might not even get won't help my healing. I'm a mass of positive thoughts and dread, and then I remember all the prayer letters I've received from several small churches. Prayers to counteract the dread and fear.

Before we leave the house, I write, *Johanna being organized, good weather for driving to chemo, decent sleep, phone call from Angie, prayer letters.*

Dr. L's very kind nurse leads us back to the exam room with a weigh-in first. I'm still under my regular weight but climbing back into reasonable. This does not make me happy, but it makes the nurse very chipper. Positive thought. Dread.

My orientation nurse suggested that I eat whatever I want whenever I want because people tend to lose weight on chemo. I'd like to stay thin just this once in my life, but I know now that unexplained weight loss is one of the clearest signs you have cancer. This is so odd to me; I gained two tumors, one in my colon and one in my liver, but instead of making me heavier, they made me lighter. Were they eating up good stuff? Did they suck up all the fat in my food and make it dissipate? I should probably do some research, but all I know is that for one full year, I was a skinny girl. How shallow am I that I wish things would stay that way?

After the weigh-in, there is the checking of my vitals and the list of questions about the meds I'm on. The suggestion has been that I bring in all my meds so they can be reviewed. One more thing to carry around—a baggy full of hydrocodone, Ambien, iron pills, Prilosec, antibiotics for a UTI that I somehow developed, and any other supplement or pill I'm taking. Instead, Johanna sat at the computer last night and created a list. Turns out I'm taking a lot of stuff. No wonder I'm gaining weight.

My blood pressure is uncharacteristically high. I've always hovered at 90 over 60, but suddenly I'm in the 135 over 95 range. It will climb in the months to come, and I'll learn that another side effect of chemo can be elevated blood pressure. There are rules in chemo land, and the big one is that anytime my top number is over 150, I can't be hooked up to the chemo drip. There will be one time when my blood pressure is 149 over 110. High for me, and I'll get hooked up, but with an admonition to try to calm down.

These are all easy things for a medical professional to say, but I wonder how they expect you to calm down when you have stage IV cancer and you're about to get pumped full of chemicals. When you're worrying about your kids and your parents and your bank account and your clients who are just being nice and allowing you to keep doing their online marketing even when your brain doesn't work very well. Dread. Positive thoughts. Prayer.

Dr. L comes in and spends a decent amount of time talking to us. The good news is that after only one treatment, my tumor marker has dropped from 81 to 65. This means everything is working the way it should. This is the news we needed to hear. I post the good results on Facebook, and in about thirty seconds, I have dozens of likes and comments. Zach's buddy Thom comments, "Hell, yeah! I feel bad for the cancer that has to go toe to toe with you, Bunny. Keep up the fight!" By evening, there will be hundreds of likes and comments, all of which are loving and kind and encouraging.

This is what keeps me sane. From the beginning, I have been open about my diagnosis and treatment. The only way I can make sense of having cancer is if I can get my community involved and hear their feedback and encouragement. If my story makes it easier for someone else someday, maybe this crazy experience will make the tiniest bit of sense. There isn't a reason I got cancer, but I have to make it work in my life. I have to find a path to sanity about this ugliness.

We go to the chemo suite, ready to take on the world with the good news. Johanna and I sign in and find a chair on the east side of the suite with a sliver of a view of the mountains and wait, a bit breathlessly, to see who is assigned to me. It is the young brunette nurse with the thick hair, not Scary Nurse. There is relief all around, and then there is the process. I know this is only my second treatment, but I'm starting to feel like an old hand.

My tumor markers are down. This week's treatment will be slightly shorter than last week's. Jennifer is coming later in the day to give Johanna a break. I didn't get Scary Nurse.

Life is pretty good right this minute, even in the chemo suite. I don't know if the gratitude is helping with the healing, but I know the good news is helping with the gratitude. I have a lot to be thankful for right this minute.

CHAPTER 23

Christmas, Canyon Road, and Overindulgence

~~→

Johanna and I had the perfect Christmas Eve with church and a Canyon Road walk with Jeanne, who treated us to a meal at Julia at La Posada downtown, which was possibly the best meal either of us had ever eaten. I frequently think that while Johanna is essential to this battle, and Jennifer is our behind-the-scenes mainstay, Jeanne is the frosting on the cake. And yes, even with cancer, a lot of my life feels like cake.

On days when Johanna and I are starting to get sick of each other, Jeanne, who seems to be in Santa Fe for the long haul, will call and say, "Let's try lunch at Casa Chimayó, guys!" or, "There's a big sale at Coldwater Creek. Let's see what good thing we can find in those old-lady racks." There is a lunch or a dinner somewhere almost every other day, and when I reach for my wallet, she always says, "Don't even think about it." She has no idea what a gift she is giving me. While I write for her birthing centers, she brings an ease to my life that is both unexpected and a relief every day. I ask her when she is headed home to Austin and she says, "Heck, those birthing centers practically run themselves. I've left the midwives in charge so that I can hang out here and boss you around."

Christmas Eve was no exception. She had guests flying in on Christmas Day, but she set aside Christmas Eve for us. The Canyon Road Walk was exactly what I wanted for my first Santa Fe Christmas. It was chilly, but not brutally cold, and we did it all — stepping into well-lit galleries, stopping on the sidewalks at little luminaria bonfires to drink hot chocolate, grabbing a hot buttered rum at El Farol from the outdoor bartender. The sky was lit with stars. At one point, it started to snow and the flakes fell into the farolitos, sizzling as they hit the candle flame. Groups sang carols, and as we passed, we joined in.

My last chemo was on the 19th, so I wasn't tired. I got to have Christmas Eve with almost no fatigue.

On Christmas Day, Johanna and I slept late. I felt better every day as I got further and further from the last chemo treatment. I made coffee and started a fire in the wood-burning stove, going outside into the crisp air to gather a pile of logs. Johanna came out of her room, hair mussed and sleepy-eyed. She hugged me, saying, "Merry Christmas, Mom. I am so happy to be here with you this morning."

Johanna's one of few words. She is an observer and takes her time before she reacts or chooses what she's going to say. She's been this way since she was a child and I used to think she was just wary. Now I know she has a discerning spirit, that she knows and sees things most of us miss because we hurtle headlong into situations. When she offers words, they mean something. Hearing her say this was Christmas present enough for me.

There were gifts under the aluminum tree, and she turned on the color wheel so it squeaked just like it did when I was in Mrs. Sandoval's first-grade classroom in 1966. We stumbled into the entry/library where the tree was set up, coffee mugs in our hands.

I went overboard for Johanna. I wanted this to be an extra-special Christmas, so there was a pile of gifts with her name on them: fur-lined Sorel boots for walking through the snowy sidewalks downtown, a Columbia Bugaboo jacket for skiing in January, ski gloves, and gift certificates for Ski Santa Fe. Elaborate eye-makeup palettes and a fuzzy pullover for cold mornings. There was a "Free Bates" T-shirt I ordered weeks ago from a *Downton Abbey* website and forgot about. It felt extravagant, but so deserved.

She was, as always, thoughtful in her gift giving. She gave me expensive lotion because the chemo makes my already dry skin worse than usual. There was a book, a journal, and two pairs of luxuriously fuzzy socks for cold mornings on our tile floor. There was an elaborate eye-makeup palette just like the one I bought her. She had wrapped up the movie *Lincoln* for me.

We finished the presents, and Johanna gathered up the trash while I boiled water for another pot of coffee in the French press. We had chocolate croissants from Chocolate Maven. We talked about going to Del Charro later. We watched the *TODAY* show and talked about other Christmases, going to Logan, skiing, and our tickets to *Les Miserables* for this afternoon. We talked about last night on Canyon Road, the music at church, and the dinner with Jeanne.

It was Christmas Day. We didn't talk about cancer.

The next day, we'd pack and go to Logan for six days. I was determined not to think about the Logan trip. I dreaded the crowds and the hot, stuffy rooms, but mostly I dreaded people crowding around, wanting physical contact, asking questions. I hadn't been home since my diagnosis. I felt certain I was facing a crush of good wishes. And instead of being pleased, I was tired thinking about it.

My plan was to be grateful, gracious, and positive all the time. In reality, I wanted to be left alone. I had always been the most social person in any group, but cancer had changed that.

I talked to my friend Angie about it. "You just don't want people all up in your business," she said in her Mississippi accent. She had moved to Logan to marry a local boy and found it to be both charming and stifling at the same time. And she was right. My business these days was cancer and it was bad enough without having to share it with everyone else. When I thought about this trip to Logan, I felt nothing other than dread.

The Christmas Day plan was to have Chinese food at Yin Yang for lunch and go to the movies. Then late in the evening, we'd go to Del Charro for our holiday green chile chowder and maybe a margarita.

I wrote in the red notebook before we went out for lunch: *Christmas in Santa Fe, Zach and Lesley calling early this morning, Lesley and the baby healthy, a day with my girl, going to the movies, life right now.* For the first time in a while, writing those lines didn't feel like something I was forcing myself to do.

CHAPTER 24

Reluctant Rock Star

~~→

We're in Logan, and I am doing my best to be sweet to everyone who stops by my parents' house to see me. All my close family is here, including my California nieces with their three little boys. It's nice, especially for my mom, who thrives on piles of people to care for. There are a lot of hugs and I tend to always have a small child on my lap, which I like. It's still exhausting. Mom, as sweet and kind as she has ever been, hovers, wanting to be sure I've eaten and that I'm not overdoing it. I know if Johanna were the sick one, I'd be a wreck. I try to be as patient as possible, but sometimes I have to get in the car and drive down to the real estate office to get away from all the attention.

The office is not much better. The first time Johanna and I escape there, a blue Dodge pickup pulls into the drive right behind us. Sabrina's dad, Lloyd, gets out and stops me before I can go in the door.

"Bunny Tewwy," he calls out, using his pet name for me, which is what I called myself in second grade. "You haven't been to see me yet!" He envelops me in his Lloyd bear hug. Lloyd was my closest neighbor and a frequent dinner/drink pal for Last Boyfriend and me when I lived here. I love Lloyd. He's family, even though he technically isn't.

Johanna smirks. "She has a really long list of social engagements this week, Lloyd. She's like the Queen of England or something."

He laughs. "Aw, hell, she always thought she was the Queen of England."

We go inside. Lloyd gets a cup of coffee and sits at my desk. There are smiles and greetings all around, and T. J. and Robin give me the latest real estate news. But first there is the requisite, "How are you feeling, what's next, what does the doctor say?" from Lloyd. T. J., Robin, and Johanna can answer him — they have all the news I have — but he wants to hear from my own lips that I'm feeling fine and things are progressing as they should.

As Lloyd is leaving, Rachel from the grocery store pulls up. T. J. raises his eyebrows and Johanna says, "Like I said, it's like she's a rock star, but without the talent or the money." T. J. laughs.

"I should make you park your car out back if I plan to get any work done."

But this is two days after Christmas, and nothing is going to happen in the Logan real estate market. So mostly we visit, and I get on the computer and relax somewhat between locals stopping by to hug me and give me their best wishes.

I love Logan and that people are so caring, but I am relieved that I live elsewhere. When I go to the Annex later in the day to celebrate December birthdays, the table is inundated with people stopping by to hug and wish me well. Someone raises an eyebrow and says, "Are you supposed to be drinking?" and I am reminded of how intrusive folks tend to be when they think they know you well.

"No one deserves a drink more," Shelley says, and I send her a grateful look. She and Larry have been through all this with Larry's colon cancer. She's one of my strongest allies.

The benefit is in three days and preparations continue in earnest. Glena and Sabrina got online and sent out emails to all the folks I know from our years going to the Atlanta and New York wholesale gift markets. Boxes arrive daily at the office. Gil from Lothantique sends a big box of luxury bath and skin-care products from Toronto. Language Art sends wall hangings from Chicago. Gaura Tibbets from Couleur Nature sends a beautiful throw made from old saris, and Erin Smith Art from Atlanta sends a canvas that I want to keep for myself. Donna from Johnny Loves June in Baton Rouge sends beautiful leather and pearl jewelry. Glenda Gies calls from Philadelphia and says a Glenda bag is on the way, but she's worried it won't arrive in time, so someone is picking one up from one of her vendors in Clovis. The Glenda bag promises to be a big-ticket item; every woman in six counties wants one.

Susan from Grandmother's Buttons in Louisiana sends two necklaces and a pair of earrings. Barbara Edelman, someone I don't know very well, sends several pieces of jewelry from Santa Fe, and I remember that she and I met once at a New York show.

I am overwhelmed by people's generosity. I read once that you should be able to sum your life up in one sentence. Right now, I feel like my sentence should be, "I knew a lot of really generous people."

Zachary is coming for the benefit on Saturday night. To surprise me, Johanna called him and said that she thought the one thing I wanted for Christmas was for him to be here, so he'll fly from Dallas to Amarillo and drive over for the night. I'm thrilled about that and would be even happier if Lesley could come as well. But they've been traveling for the holidays already, and she's a pregnant girl trying to keep my grandson healthy.

I know I will forever be in debt to the people who did all the hard work and made the benefit happen. The money and the spirit of love it created will make all the difference in my life for the hard months of recovery to come.

I write this later on CaringBridge, after the first of the year:

Last Saturday night, an entire cast of people who care about me and my family put together and executed a benefit for me that was overwhelming in a dozen ways—by the people who worked, the crowd that attended, the meal that was served, the items that were donated, the money that was raised, and most of all, by the love and kindness that permeated every corner of the room.

I have a lot of good memories from the evening: Glena, Sabrina, Anna Lee, Shelley, and Raynee in the serving line, dipping green or red chile over the flat enchiladas provided by Warren and Angie and the Annex; my brother, Klee, and my best Albuquerque pal, Bruce, standing together, visiting behind auction items; my niece, Kyla, and cousin, Tim, fighting over the Michael Rohner hummingbird print in the auction; me getting to visit with folks I haven't seen in months, or even years; my great-nieces and nephews all sitting together at one table; Kene and Bruce playing guitar together at the dance; Zach and Johanna in the midst of everything, and through it all, T. J. overseeing all the workers and making sure everything ran smoothly.

In just a few hours, you guys raised almost $17,000, a crazy number, especially for a small town of less than 1,100 people, most of whom are on a fixed budget. It's a testament to what people can do when they all come together for a specific cause. It's also a testament to how small towns work. We may get accused of being meddlesome gossips, but when push comes to shove, my hometown takes good care of its own. I'm proud to be a part of that very hard-working, caring community.

Words are inadequate for how I feel about the benefit and people's responses to my needs. Let me just say that for every low I had in 2012, I had three or four highs, and those continue.

Happy New Year. I'm grateful for all of you. Thanks for checking in.

CHAPTER 25

Prognosis: Twelve Months

～➤

It's January. A new year with new worries, a new deductible to pay, new chemo treatments coming up. I continue to agonize over my financial situation. One would think that I spend my time thinking about my health, about recovery, about the damn cancer, but the truth is that I mostly think about money.

"You have that $250,000 life insurance policy," T. J. says, because in addition to being my cousin and my supporter-deluxe, he is also my insurance guy. "If you want, you're allowed to cash it in and get a portion of that money to live on, especially when you have a life-threatening condition. You could probably get about $115,000."

I seem to have a life-threatening condition these days.

"You just have to get your oncologist to write a letter telling the insurance company what your prognosis is."

At my next appointment, which seems to follow too closely on the heels of the last appointment, Dr. L goes through my blood tests and tells me I'm good for my third chemo treatment on Wednesday. I bring up the letter to the insurance company.

"Sure," Dr. L says. "I write those all the time. What exactly do you need for it to say?"

"I guess the truth. Right?"

"Right. I can't make something up. But how specific do you need for me to be? And do you want to see it before it gets sent?"

I tilt my head and look at him.

"Well, Bunny, people sometimes don't want to read what their prognosis is. Seeing it in black and white is sometimes a shock. I can just send it directly if you prefer."

I'm tough. Johanna's tough. We aren't going to be set back by a letter to my life insurance company.

"Nah," I say, "just go ahead and write it, and I'll pick it up so I can get it to T. J. to send on."

"Okay," he says and turns to the nurse. "Make a note for me to write the life insurance letter before Friday this week."

On Friday afternoon, after I'm unplugged from the pump and when I'm ready for my celebratory lunch (Yay! We've made it through our third treatment!), Johanna stops at the desk downstairs and picks up the promised letter.

"Should we open it?" she asks, and I nod.

"I know I'm going to get well. What could the big deal be?"

I read it first and then start to cry. Not a pretty cry. She takes it, reads it, and then turns to me, eyes shining, and says, "It's not the truth. This is not what's going to happen."

Here is what the letter says. After the initial explanation of my diagnosis: "51-year-old female, Metastatic colon cancer with a corresponding 4.5-cm lesion on the liver..." etc. Then there is a line that reads, "Based on medical findings, patient's prognosis is 12 months."

We are quiet on the drive home. I know we need the celebratory lunch. I also know we need the life insurance money. But I know we will never send that letter to anyone. It is not true. It cannot be true. It will not be true.

CHAPTER 26
Bad Cancer Bitch

~~>

Today was not a great day. This is an off week, which meant no chemo last Wednesday, so I wasn't too tired to go to church. Chemo weeks are tired weeks, exhausted-be-yond-belief weeks. I sometimes make it to church on chemo weeks, but not often.

I like church now. It's a shock to me sometimes, after all those years at home when my parents made all of us go to the Baptist Church every time the door was opened, three times a week. Or those years when my kids were little and my mom would call to see if we had made it to church that morning—not necessarily guilting me into going, but making me feel like all the really good moms had their kids in Sunday School that day.

Now I love going. Christ Church, my friends there, the light through the window above the pulpit, the music, the sermons. The love and grace. I never knew a relationship with God and a church community could be about grace and love instead of anger and fear and dread.

Martin prayed at church for a dozen things, some celebra-tory and some not. At one point, he said, "And Lord, I pray for those of us who are having to run a race we did not choose to run." This morning I wanted to run away from my life. At that moment I wanted to tear the number from my jersey and stop running the race, stop being the optimistic one who was writing all the cheerful CaringBridge posts about the link between cancer and gratitude. I was tired of being the center of everyone's attention. I was tired of being sick.

There is a man at church whose name I don't recall. Chemo brain is real and besides, I'm not very interested in getting to know a lot of new people right now. That lack of interest is not like me, but nothing about this life is like me right now.

We've been introduced before, and from the church network or prayer chain or something, he knows my story. He came up to me today to discuss, of course, cancer. He was quick to tell me a long, involved story about his daughter having some sort of cancer that resulted in a life-threatening blood loss, weeks of ICU, and then chemo treatment. His story went on for a long time, and I kept thinking, "Is there some reason you think I want to hear the story of your child's cancer disaster?" This wasn't the day I wanted him to share this tale. I hated to be selfish, but all I could think was, "I have cancer. This doesn't make me feel better, and I think you're all supposed to be in the business of making me feel better." Being at church didn't make me feel better today.

In the middle of hopefully the end of his story, this man's son — not the bad cancer disaster child but a marginally handsome man in at least his late thirties — walked up, and the storyteller whispered, "Oh, and I have been so wanting to introduce my son to your daughter." I looked at his son, who was the same age as my last boyfriend, and then I looked at my beautiful twenty-two-year-old daughter. I wanted to kick both men, or turn away from them, or say, "Have you seen my girl? She's Anne Hathaway or Natalie Portman, but prettier. And smarter. Your son will not be introduced to my daughter."

I was a bad cancer bitch today, which is what I am some days. It's never the plan, but frequently, I end up wanting to bite someone's head off. I don't even know what my life is about anymore. I frequently say a prayer that goes something like, "Please, please, please let me be nice to people today." It doesn't always work, but I continue to pray for that.

I left the house in the middle of the afternoon and went downtown to Collected Works Bookstore near the plaza. I wasn't sure I needed to buy any books, but I needed to get out of the house, where said beautiful daughter was watching *Live from the Red Carpet* on E!, leading up to the Golden Globe Awards. I couldn't wrap my brain around four or five hours of watching Ryan Seacrest admire evening gowns. Johanna had responded to a couple of questions in a short and sarcastic (at least to me) tone. Instead, I went out in the 19-degree weather, saying I was going to the bookstore and the grocery store.

She offered, in a desultory fashion, to go with me, but I was sick of both of us and determined to get out of my dark, somewhat cold home, where the only warmth was on the couch in front of the television. "No," I said, "I'm good, and I just want to check out some new titles at the bookstore."

I don't drive much these days. The weeks I have chemo are hard and I'm lightheaded. Johanna reminds me that I'm taking a lot of Ambien, which creates a whole new set of cognitive issues. When I finally feel like it, driving is almost a gift. Just driving the seven blocks to Collected Works should be a treat. Except that nothing is going to be a treat today, it seems.

I find a parking place across from Collected Works, always a small miracle in downtown Santa Fe, and without warning, I lean my forehead against the steering wheel and begin to sob. I feel bad for the man with the daughter with cancer, and I feel bad for Martin, having to be the shepherd when most of us are so obviously floundering, and I really feel bad for myself, being the cancer bitch with no relief in sight. But mostly I cry for Johanna, for her life being put on hold in this last semester of college, when she should be spending her Sunday afternoons either in the UNM library, studying or at a friend's house, watching the damnable red carpet, or in a sports bar drinking beer and watching a football game. She says over and over that she wants to be here and nowhere else, but her saying it doesn't make it right that at twenty-two, she is the caregiver for someone with stage IV cancer. She should be having fun. I know I'm not a lot of fun most days. My heart is broken for her.

She will be going to Wisconsin in a few weeks to stay several days with Jason, and when I think of her being gone, I'm panicked. We planned the Wisconsin trip around my chemo treatments. She will leave early on a Friday morning, while I'm still on the pump but done with my in-house treatment. My sister and two cousins will arrive to haul me around in my post-pump lightheaded and tired state. Because it is a weekend in Santa Fe for them, we will go shopping and out to dinner and for drinks, when all I'll want is to be sitting at home with a book and Johanna.

When I think of someone besides Johanna being in the house with me, I feel sick. While my heart is broken for her, I can't stand the thought of being without her. I can't stand the thought of getting up in the morning without her sleeping in the next room.

I am an emotional mess. I can't stop being selfish while I can't bear her having to be in charge right now. She has said several times, "Mom, if I get a cold, someone else will have to come and take care of you." I'm supposed to be the person who takes care of her, not the other way around. I was the strongest, healthiest person I knew in the entire world. How did this get to be my life? And hers?

I make myself get out of the car and go into Collected Works. I suspect that a room full of books and a seat next to the fireplace will make me feel better. I find Stegner's *Crossing to Safety* and a chick-lit piece I've considered getting on my Kindle for a while. And then I see Larry McMurtry's *Last Picture Show* and have to pick it up, even if I've read it eight or ten or twelve times. In fact, I read it just a month ago, but now I can't think where my copy is, so I just buy another one. I can't remember anything anymore, and I've taken to being very self-indulgent with myself.

At home I am deep into Doug Preston's *Cities of Gold*, which I love most of the time. But my brain is so foggy and the book is so thick that I'm finding it difficult to focus. I need to read something I've already read a dozen times. I need not to think.

This book comforts me like an old friend. I get a cup of coffee, sit near the fire, and start the McMurtry book, reading a few of the opening pages. I think of the first time I read this book back when Zachary was a baby, the two of us in that tiny house in West Texas while Harold was out on the tractor. It made me think of my uncles running the movie house in San Jon, New Mexico, in the '40s and '50s. When I read it in West Texas, I had no idea what my life would become. And here I am.

Thinking about Zachary makes me feel better. Thinking about him and Lesley making a place for my new grandson is comforting. Johanna will graduate from college this May, and there will be a baby boy here for the graduation. I can get well for that. I know I can.

I have three days until my next chemo treatment. Usually, these are the days I feel the best physically, the days when my nose stops running all the time and my eyes stop watering and my mouth stops tasting like it's filled with angry metal. The diarrhea subsides somewhat. I start to get my appetite back, and I have more energy right at the end. I have only one bloody nose per day instead of four or five. My taste buds recover, and a glass of wine tastes okay. If only my emotions recovered in the same way.

I pay for the three books, including the McMurtry, knowing that somewhere at home, buried in one of my stacks, I probably also have a copy of the Stegner, but I don't know where. Chemo brain is very real. I feel old and tired most days, and my brain always feels old and tired.

After sitting among all those books and having a cup of coffee, I suddenly want to get back to Johanna and the Golden Globes. We are sure *Les Miserables* will win everything, but we feel hopeful for Ben Affleck and *Argo*. Just sitting on the red couch with her will make me feel better. Tomorrow's another day.

That evening in the red notebook, I write, *Collected Works, Stegner and McMurtry, Argo winning, Martin and church, Johanna.* It is what I have right now, and I'm grateful. Not small stuff.

Chapter 27
Bone Tired

~~>

I'm bone tired in a way I've never been before. Even when Johanna was a tiny, unhappy, colicky baby, I wasn't this tired. Even when I was a single mom, all alone, and I had to get up and go to work after caring for her through the night, or after helping Zach with a project that took us until midnight to complete. And "bone" tired is the right description. My bones ache with exhaustion. I think I can feel the poison seeping through them. There are aches I've never had before.

This is what Sarah was talking about when she described how worn out chemo makes you feel. "You lie on the couch and tell yourself you need to go to the bathroom, and an hour later, you tell yourself the same thing, but you won't be able to make your legs hit the floor and stand up. You'll be too tired. Lifting your head will be too much," she said.

That's how I feel. My head is too heavy for my neck to hold it up. I can't even lift the laptop some days. Johanna hands it to me without speaking, knowing I don't have the wherewithal to pick it up.

Chemo sucks in a lot of ways but feeling this worn out is one of the worst. Not only am I physically beat up, but I can't get my thoughts together. I lie on the red couch and watch hours of television because I can't concentrate enough to read a book. I might as well forget about writing anything for any of my clients. I have no words and no creative energy. I feel empty.

I don't even want to log onto Facebook, which is where I get most of my encouragement. Everyone is behind me 100 percent, or so I hear. My posts are always at the top of the page because I get so many responses. On the days when I post something about my cancer and the treatment and how I'm feeling, I'm the most popular person online.

I never post the negative stuff. I never complain on Facebook, or out there in the world. Someday I know I will have to apologize to Johanna because she is the only person who gets the darkest part of me, the whining and the impossible food cravings and the almost daily reluctance to get out of bed or off the couch. I do my best to make sure no one knows about the bad days, other than Johanna. And maybe Jeanne and Jennifer.

I wonder about other people I've known who did well with cancer. Surely they had dark days like this as well. T. J. also gets some of that darkness when he calls each day to check on me, on us. He'll ask, "How's it going?" and when I hesitate, he'll say, "Not so good today?"

I'll affirm that the day is marginal, and I'll extract a promise from him that he will not pass that along to anyone other than Robin. I picture the real estate office in Logan with people coming in and out, asking about me. He says traffic has picked up because everyone stops by to see what my daily news is. Locals know that he and my parents are talking to me on a regular basis. Best of all, locals know that if they're going to bother anyone with questions, it's better all the way around if they bug T. J. rather than my parents.

He asks and I let out a sigh. He agrees to tell everyone that things aren't perfect but that I'm doing pretty well, considering that it's only the second day since I got off the pump. What he and I both know is that this is the absolute worst day of the cycle. On the pump, I've got two days of steroids to keep me going and to ramp up my appetite.

During orientation, Joyce the Nurse said the steroids were great motivators, that they made patients feel so good that they spent those days doing all their housework. I haven't had that feeling, but I do know that the steroids make a difference in my appetite. And, of course, they make it impossible to sleep. Like in the '80s, when I tried speed a time or two, the steroids make me lie awake at night with my eyes wide open and my heart racing. But unlike the '80s, I'm tired underneath the crazy, revved-up heart rate. Bone tired.

I lie on the couch and watch *Big Bang Theory* reruns with Johanna or *Keeping Up with the Kardashians*, although I made her promise she wouldn't reveal that to anyone. Sunday nights are good because we have *Downton Abbey* to look forward to. And *Game of Thrones*. We have Xfinity on Demand, and we're addicted to *New Girl* and *The Mindy Project*. I've never watched so much television in my entire life.

We've become sedentary animals for these winter days while I'm on the pump and the three days after. I get disconnected on a Friday. Generally, it's Monday before I want to move. I try to get showered and put together for church on Sunday morning, although never for the early service. I struggle to make it to church. After we arrive, we say hello to everyone who wants to give us hugs and encouragement. When we finally get seated and there's standing and sitting for songs and prayers, I end up sitting. Standing makes me dizzy. Standing for too long makes my vertigo from the middle of the night return.

And church makes me cry. I know that's mostly because being so tired makes me emotional. But there are also the moments when Martin says something before prayers such as, "And if the battles life is presenting are too much for you today…," and I'm immediately in tears. I'm fighting a battle I didn't choose, I'm exhausted, and I'm trying to act as though I'm sure what the outcome will be. I spend an inordinate amount of energy convincing the universe that I know I'm going to win this battle, that I'm certain it's only a matter of time before it's all over and I'm healthy again. But I'm not. I'm not certain.

I work on the gratitude piece. I write in the red notebook, and I talk to my parents. They spent a few days here recently and took me to my doctor's visit and to my chemo. I wanted them to see that it's all going well. Having them here was a comfort. Johanna is so busy with the beginning of her last semester of college that it made sense for all of us to have them in charge Monday through Thursday. I was buoyed up by their help, by my dad taking the car in for an oil change, by my mom cooking chicken and dumplings and scrubbing my toilets. And by their attitude that as long as we're all together, everything will be fine.

But then it was Wednesday, and I had chemo. And then it was Thursday, and I was revved up on steroids. They headed home, seeing me with so much energy. Not house-cleaning energy, but energy nonetheless.

Now it's Sunday, and I've been disconnected from the pump for forty-eight hours. My head is foggy, and I can't get off the couch. I can't think of a thing to write in the red notebook because I can't think of a thing, period. I'm just tired.

CHAPTER 28

Am I Even a Candidate?

From the first meeting with Dr. L, the goal has been to get well. But what that really means is that the goal has been to get my tumors shrunk enough to have surgery. I can't survive with the tumors intact for the long haul. They have to go.

I have brought up the surgery option on occasion, just for fun (and out of fear). His standard reply has been, "You're doing very well. Your tumors are reacting exactly how we want them to. The 5FU is working. Let's give it a little more time."

Before a treatment in January, which is treatment number four overall, he says, "I want to send your records to my associate, Dr. C, at MD Anderson. He's the master at liver surgery, and that's what you need. He can take a look, and he'll decide whether he wants an appointment with you or not."

Wait! I think. *After all this, I might not even get an appointment with the surgeon?* The minute Johanna and I are out of the room with Dr. L, I post on Facebook. "My records are going to the MD Anderson surgeon. Everyone send up their best prayers and good thoughts that he accepts me for a consult."

I don't add that I also need prayers that he'll then think I'm a good candidate for surgery. Our lives are so dependent on the hope that I can have surgery. I don't dare put out there that I have any doubts. Yes, Dr. C will see me. Yes, Dr. C will think I'm a good candidate for surgery.

There is so much happening all at once. My hair is starting to thin, which is one of the side effects my orientation nurse talked about. It's always been a well-known fact that you not only get the most dreaded of all diseases, but you also lose your hair. The crazy thing is that when it happens to you, that first pillow covered with hair is a surprise. Initially you thought, *not me!* when you heard the word *cancer*. And then you thought it again when the doctor suggested chemo. One would think that when the hair starts to pile up on the bathroom floor, you'd be resigned to what's happening, but you're still thinking, *Not me!*

Besides every chemo treatment getting progressively harder to take (with the bleeding gums and the ongoing, somewhat uncontrollable diarrhea), in the midst of all this, I'm talking to a really cute guy on OkCupid. I have no idea why. I know I'm never going to have a real meet and greet with him, but I just like the idea. It's a sweet distraction to anxiously scan my emails to see if I have a notification that he messaged me. I lie in bed thinking about how much fun a late-night conversation on the phone with someone sweet and intelligent and interesting would be. I don't even think about sex anymore. My port is still as ugly as it was in the beginning. I've started gaining weight and I'm starting to puff up with all the steroids I take every other week. They make my cheeks rosy, but my skinny jeans tight.

Honestly. Whoever thought up this system should be fired.

Luckily the guy I'm emailing is going to California for a couple of weeks to visit family. He's allegedly a writer and a therapist, and the emails I get are fun and playful. I've written on my profile that my one life goal is to visit all the Major League Baseball stadiums in the nation, and he and I list the ones we've visited. I say I want to go to San Francisco and spend one evening in the stands and one in the bay in a kayak, waiting on a home run to come over the top of the outfield fence.

"I've done that!" he says, delighted that someone else gets it. He launches into a description of exactly the kind of evening I want in my life somewhere down the road. We compare notes on Coors Field and figure out that once, a couple of years ago, we were probably there at the same time. Of course, he was probably with a date and I was with Last Boyfriend, so we wouldn't have done very well at a meet and greet, but still. Some parts of these emails are feeling like something akin to hope.

"When I get back from Cali, let's get together. Let's go to CCA and catch a movie," he writes. I think, *oh well, maybe I'll get brave enough to do something like that.* Hell, I'm fighting cancer. What's the worst thing that could happen on a date with a stranger who writes such beautiful emails? And he's a distraction from the hair on my pillow. I try not to feel guilty about the deception.

What I don't know yet is that when he presses for a meet and greet and I tell him about the cancer, he'll go radio silent. I'll never hear another word from him again. But I'll understand. Who would want to date the woman with the thin hair and the ugly port?

On January 31, I get a call from a number I don't recognize.

"Ms. Terry?" the caller says. "This is Lakeshia from MD Anderson. I'm Dr. C's scheduling supervisor. I'd like to talk to you about coming in for a consult with him."

I want to shout, even though I'm on day six after treatment and still feeling washed out. "Yes, yes," I say breathlessly, "tell me how it works."

"Well, Ms. Terry, I'm going to send you an email with a set of instructions and records we still need. But let's tentatively set you up for February 18 to meet with Dr. C."

We talk for a few more minutes, and I get off the phone. "Johanna!" I shout down the hall to where she's working on a paper. "Johanna! We are going to Houston!"

For one entire minute, I don't think about the cost, about being cut open, about pain or fear or anything remotely unpleasant. She comes into the room and I grab her hands and start to dance. "We are going to Houston!" and she smiles with me. "Cool. I've never been to Houston before!"

CHAPTER 29

Houston

∿➤

It's Saturday. I had chemo on Wednesday, got off the pump on Friday, and tomorrow, Johanna and I will board a plane to Houston. The benefit money is still holding out. I've spent hours on the internet, trying to find a reasonably priced place for us to stay. MD Anderson emails their patients a list of lodging options that offer medical discounts, but when you call, the answer is, "Yes, we mark our $185 business rate down to $159 per night." We will be there three nights and, as always, we are on a very tight budget.

Every review I read says something about how the lodger had to be in town for several weeks for a medical procedure. My kind of people.

I'm optimistic. Yes, I have cancer. I'm in the middle of a chemo regimen. I feel like shit 90 percent of the time. But still, this feels like progress.

I'll be seeing Dr. C, one of Dr. L's superiors when he was training at MD Anderson. When I asked if I could have this surgery in Albuquerque, Dr. L said, "You know, liver surgery is tricky. I want you to see the best guy there is..." and trailed off. I didn't know liver surgery was any trickier than any other kind of surgery. The things I don't know.

When I sent out a prayer request to the Wine-Drinking Bible Study Girls about this trip, Kristi emailed me back. "Great news! Dr. C was my mom's surgeon."

It is great news. Her mom, Doris, had colon cancer ten years ago that mirrored mine, and I vaguely knew that a surgeon had removed something like 60 percent of her liver. Doris is now cancer-free and never slows down. She has eleven grandchildren all over New Mexico and she travels around to take care of them. She helps run the ranch in Roy, New Mexico. If Doris can do this, maybe I can.

Doris calls me later in the day after she hears from Kristi. She has a high, sweet voice, and I'm happy to hear from her. I recently sent her a thank-you note for cash she and her husband, Ray, sent me when I was diagnosed.

"Bunny, I'm so excited that you're seeing Dr. C! We love him, love him, love him." Her voice sings over the wire. Doris and Ray live on a ranch in the Canadian River Canyon. It's a ranch that's been in the Hartley family for more than one hundred years. In the '90s, it was a dude ranch where tourists from places like Germany, Japan, and India came to help with the branding. For crazy amounts of money, they paid to help out on the ranch. They live in a beautiful part of New Mexico and I wish I was in her kitchen drinking coffee with her instead of here at my desk, trying to book a room near the Texas Medical Center for less than $120 per night.

She tells me that of course he'll accept me as a patient, that he's smart and ambitious, and that he hates cancer as much as we do. "And he's a very good-looking man," Doris says, and I smile. Doris is the mother of our Amy, who is married to my nephew, Kene. I am the best aunt in the world to Kene and Amy's little girls. And I trust Doris to give me the scoop. We are all in a big circle of love and family, and I trust that love to sustain me.

I'm doing that a lot these days.

I ask her about recovery time and for tricks for getting ready for major abdominal surgery. I already had this conversation with Larry last week, during which he and Shelley scared the shit out of me.

"It's going to hurt like hell. There's just no other way to say it," Larry said, with Shelley nodding in agreement. Larry and I go way back. Our parents went to high school together. His little sister was one of my best buddies as a child. We went on summer vacations together when I was a kid, flying trips to Tres Ritos in the mountains of northern New Mexico when it rained so heavily that our farmer daddies couldn't work in the fields. He was my cousin David's best friend and roommate right after high school, when they decided they were going to be Quay County farming buddies. And then he married my best friend from high school.

I trust Larry. I know he won't sugarcoat anything. He knows all the hard facts. He's gone under the knife four or five times to manage his colon cancer and other complications, but now he is cancer-free.

Damn cancer. Damn surgery. But wow, to get to hear the words *cancer-free*.

Larry recommended several things. "Get a walker and a toilet extender. You're not going to believe how much it hurts just to sit down and get up from the toilet. Your ab muscles will be split in two. Hell, Bunny, rolling over in bed will make you want to cry." He went on to tell me that what the surgeon does is cut you open, take your colon out of your body, and lay it on a table beside you.

"No way!" I say. This is sounding medieval.

"Yeah. You'll hurt in ways you won't believe. You don't realize it now, but you use those stomach muscles for everything."

Shelley recommended that I buy clothes that won't touch my belly. "You know how irritating scars can be. And it's going to be healing for a really long time." She told me to buy a lot of extra-large pajama pants and dresses that hang loosely on my body. She says I won't want even my underwear touching the incision.

Larry says to get up and walk at the first opportunity. "Not that it will be a problem. Those nurses will have you up on your feet almost immediately. They'll be damn near cruel about it."

I'm scared, but grateful. So many people talk in nebulous terms when what you want are hard, concrete facts that you can process on your own. It reminds me of when I was pregnant and wanted to know real facts about birth instead of hearing about how the glow of childbirth erases the memory of pain. I wanted to know how an episiotomy healed and how contractions felt, but what I heard was, "Oh, it'll be over sooner than you think" and, "In a month, you won't even remember how it felt." I went on to have a hard thirty-six-hour labor with Zachary, cussing those glowing tales the entire time.

Getting real facts about surgery from Larry and Shelley is like a gift. Kind of like a gift with a rattlesnake in the bottom of the box, but still a gift. If I know the rattlesnake is there, I can figure out a way to handle it.

None of this good information will matter if my liver tumors are in the wrong place. If I'm not a good candidate for the surgery, I can basically come home to Santa Fe, have the tumor in my colon removed, and try to fight the liver lesions some other way. That's what Sarah is doing right now, trying to get treated by a doctor in Denver who will plant radioactive seeds near her liver lesions. It's a controversial new treatment and not proven, but when you have lesions scattered like buckshot throughout your liver, you take what you can get. That's what she says.

What I want is to have the scheduled blood tests and CT scan and my consult at MD Anderson ASAP. Suddenly, that ASAP is here. I'm so grateful. I write in the red notebook, *Benefit cash, call from Doris, Shelley and Larry, my clients who keep sending me work even though my brain doesn't work well, prayers from the Wine-Drinking Bible Study Group.* Today I have a lot to be grateful for.

CHAPTER 30

If the Cancer Doesn't Kill Me

⌇➤

I'm scheduled for another CT scan. I worry about that. I have now had four CT scans in less than four months. Someone sent me an article that says I'm putting myself at risk for another type of cancer from all the radiation contained in a CT scan, which is similar to having fifty chest X-rays. Not information I needed to receive this week, but people like to think they're being helpful.

My MD Anderson tests are scheduled for an early start on Monday morning at the Mays Clinic, which is part of the huge complex that is the Texas Medical Center. Johanna and I have studied the maps and done our research on MD Anderson. I read that it is the cancer center that has the highest success rate in the nation, closely followed by Memorial Sloan Kettering in New York. The maps show blocks and blocks of Houston, with buildings like the Texas Children's Hospital, Texas Women's Center, Methodist Hospital, and Baylor Teaching Hospital all clustered close to MD Anderson and its dozen or so buildings. Wikipedia says it is the largest medical center in the world, larger than downtown Dallas. Supposedly, they treat sixty thousand patients per day there.

It's overwhelming. But I'm determined to find my way to the Mays Clinic on Monday and get my tests out of the way.

Then we'll have Tuesday free, and Johanna and I will try to find a way to entertain ourselves in a city we've never visited. Zach will drive down from Dallas on Tuesday evening and spend the night with us. Then the three of us will see Dr. C for a consult on Wednesday in the main MD Anderson building.

When did my kids get put in charge of my health care? When did this become the thing we do together? We have had fun in a thousand different ways, but this doesn't feel like fun to me. Still, I'm grateful to have them, grateful to see Zach however and whenever I can.

I'm also a mess of fear and excitement. I'm happy that Dr. C reviewed my records and accepted an appointment with me. I'm happy that my insurance has allowed this consult. I'm pleased that Doris knows him and has such positive things to say. I like having all the practical information from Larry and Shelley, scary as it is. And I'm excited to have my kids spend the night with me, just the three of us all together.

But I'm also scared to death. If I'm not a candidate for surgery, I'm screwed. If I am, I'm facing the knife and a big, ugly scar across my belly for the rest of my life. Seems like maybe the odds aren't in my favor either way.

We're headed to Houston. Dammit.

CHAPTER 31

Is There a Silver Lining?

~~→

People with cancer think about money all the time. Maybe it's only single women like me, who have been the sole providers for their households for years, but from what I can tell, people with cancer think about money all the time—how much they have, how long it will last, how much their co-pay for treatment will be next month, how much that trip to Houston for an initial visit or a follow-up will be, how they're going to keep paying the rent or the mortgage or the car payment.

I honestly don't know how it's done, except that I'm doing it. Worrying about survival, death, pain, and logistics while also thinking about cash flow all the time. And what do patients do if they have no family or friends or a benefit or maybe an employer who deems it their job to make sure you don't have to worry about money for all the time when you're laid low by the effects of the disease and treatments? I'm grateful for my support system.

The benefit money helps. Zach and Lesley pay my health insurance premium. I get random cards with checks from friends and some from people I've never met. I even get $100 bills in get-well cards, sent from West Texas (thank you, Suzanne) or northern New Mexico. One of my Mississippi cousins sent a check for $500. My ex-husband and his sweet wife are sending me their tithe every month. They tell my mom that's what they feel God wants them to do.

Jeanne takes us to lunch and dinner. People from church bring us meals. I am awash in generosity and love, and I'm grateful. But still I worry.

I run Excel spreadsheets. I have the money from the sale of my house and the money my social media management and writing provides, but when you start talking about the amounts of money that medical care takes these days, you can be wiped out overnight. What this disease means is that I'll use those funds from the sale of my house to live on, and when I want to buy my dream Santa Fe house, I won't have that nest egg. Instead of dwelling on that fact, I work on moving forward. I practice gratitude for the largess that I'm receiving from outside my own bank accounts. T.J. and Robin still send me one-third of every commission they receive. They continue to work, and I continue to try to get well, and in their most generous way, they provide me with what would be an income if I were working for them. "Shoot, Bunny," T. J. says, "you gathered up most of these clients and properties before you left, so it just makes sense."

It doesn't make sense, but I'm happy to receive those checks. It restores some of my pride to be able to say, "Well, I just got paid on a deal that's been in the works for a while."

I'm wondering how my credit will look when (if) this is over. Maybe there really is a plan. Maybe I'm being saved from a place with a roof that leaks and a tax bill that skyrockets.

I'm so clueless and bumbling most of the time. Some days, though, I feel inspired to do something about the cancer and money issues. Maybe I'll set up a nonprofit that will do things like give single moms with cancer grocery money and pay their utilities, or help with the airfare to Houston when they finally get a doctor's appointment with a surgeon, or with the hotel rooms. Houston rooms near the medical center are a damn racket. Yes, you can stay somewhere for $59 per night, but one thing you don't need when you have cancer and you're facing a consult with a guy who wants to cut your gut open is a hotel room where you have to wear your shoes in the shower. Filthy and frantic don't go together very well in my experience.

I wonder what my life will look like on the other side of this disease, when I'm well and I've used up all my resources. I didn't want to get to my mid-fifties with no money saved. I was excited when I made such a nice profit on my house and knew I had a fat chunk of cash to tide me over for the long haul. But that's rapidly disappearing.

Cancer totally sucks. And the bigger question is whether I'll get to the "other side" of this disease. I might not get well. The printed percentages for stage IV survival are not high. I'm not thinking about that today though, because I'm instead thinking about money. Perhaps the space taken up in my brain by worrying about finances is a blessing of its own.

I go back to the idea of a nonprofit. Funds for cancer patients who need them for very practical purposes. Those words run around in my head. There is the American Cancer Society. Their Santa Fe coordinator can get you reduced rates for your family when they come to visit. They'll give you a wig if your hair falls out.

There's also the Cancer Foundation for New Mexico. If you qualify, you get grocery cards, free lodging, and gas for your car. I understand from the bit of literature the social worker at the chemo center gave me that their only mission is to help people in northern New Mexico who are seeking treatment at my cancer center. But I don't qualify for their services. I have a dwindling wad of cash in the bank that disqualifies me.

There's a group called Corporate Angels, which is a network of people who fly corporate jets to different destinations and sometimes offer to take you along if you have to travel for treatment. But they don't seem to travel from Albuquerque or

Santa Fe. "Oh, no," the Corporate Angels person on the phone says. "We don't really have planes in that area." I would have been better off to get cancer in Chicago or L.A.

I need to do some research. I need to find a purpose in all this. There are people who haven't had a house sale or a benefit or a Bible study group to bring patients food every night after chemo treatments. There are people out there thinking of money all the time, all the time, all the time. Unlike me. I only think of money every other hour. I need to find a way to help those other folks as soon as I get well. I have to find a silver lining.

There is one good thing about chemotherapy: the chemical concoction makes my skin glow. I noticed it immediately. When I got up the day after my first treatment, I looked like I had a slight sunburn. I went out to the kitchen, where Johanna was toasting two pieces of bread for a peanut-butter breakfast.

"Is my face really red?" I asked her.

She turned and looked at me. "Yeah. That's totally weird, Mom. Should we call the nurse?"

It was early December, and I had many chemo treatments ahead of me. I was still hooked up to the pump and was hyper-sensitive to its whirr every ninety seconds.

"I don't know. Do I feel hot, like I have a fever?"

She laid the back of her hand against my forehead, in just the way I used to when she was little and I wanted an accurate mom-reading of a fever.

"You're a little warm."

We scrambled for the thermometer, worried about my being sick with something besides cancer, but the reading was just above normal — 99.1.

She called Joyce, the nurse on call at the Cancer Center, and left a message about my very red face and my marginal fever.

Joyce called back within ten minutes. "Nothing to worry about," she said. "It's just what the steroids do. But remember—if your temp goes over 100.1 and stays there for more than six hours, go to the emergency room."

She was right about the slight rise in temperature. What I've found in the past two months while I've had treatments is that I'm always red-faced on the days I take the steroids. I already know that the worst side effect of those particular meds is that I can't sleep very well, which leads to my taking two Ambiens instead of one, which leads to what feels like a fist fight to get extra Ambien from the doc on chemo day. Some docs see Ambien as my due, as in, "Dammit, I have cancer, and I should get whatever narcotics I need to get me through this life of chemo and chemicals." But other doctors, if Dr. L or the sweet young Dr. G are not on call, have given me a hard time about the Ambien.

But that's another story, one that involves me dissolving into an ugly-cry in the Walgreens' parking lot over a shorted prescription of Ambien because one doctor at the cancer center thinks she should monitor my Ambien usage. Why would a doctor be ugly about something that helps me sleep when sleep is so elusive? Won't I heal faster if I can sleep? You're welcome to argue narcotic addiction with me some other time. If I don't heal, I don't live, so does it really matter?

But now people remark, "Wow! Your skin looks amazing." Regardless of what is happening to most of my body, I get a dozen compliments a week on my pretty skin. The rest of this deal totally sucks, but I'll take a positive wherever I can get it. My skin looks amazing. And I'm not spending a penny on skin products. That's a silver lining I'll take any day. You have to find the light wherever you can.

Of course, there is the fact that the steroids are making me puffy. And that my hair is still thinning. What a trade. Great skin for thin hair. Something to note in the red notebook.

CHAPTER 32

Cupcakes, Wine, and a Slumber Party

～➤

We are home from Houston, road-weary and probably a bit tired of each other, but it was a productive trip. MD Anderson is impressive due to its size and efficiency. But it is also overwhelming and as crowded as the sidewalks of Manhattan. I felt like I was a cow in a feedlot, being fed through a chute into the next procedure. Not that the care wasn't good and the staff generally friendly and kind. It was just so much — and that, on top of being surrounded by really sick people and being sick myself.

The best part was that Zachary drove in from Dallas and joined the party on Tuesday evening, the night before my consult with Dr. C. The three of us had dinner in Rice Village and a couple of bottles of wine and a slumber party at the Crowne Plaza. Johanna and I bought all our favorite cupcake flavors earlier in the day — sprinkles, red velvet, sea salt and caramel, German chocolate cake, and one double-fudge chocolate. If we had to go see the cancer surgery guy, we were at least going to be self-indulgent in the process. After the great dinner and the wine, the three of us came back to the room and had more wine and split up the cupcakes.

As we were settling down after hours of talking, Zach was in the bed next to Johanna and me. After the lights went out, we kept remembering something we wanted to tell one another. After all the laughing and remembering old stories, I thought, *getting diagnosed with cancer is nearly worth it if I get to have a slumber party with my kids.* That night was a gift to my weary, worried soul, especially when we all collapsed into giggling at fart jokes, which is where all slumber parties end up.

The second-best part was finally meeting Dr. C on Wednesday morning after the grueling, long tests I underwent on Monday. Monday had been a day of tests at the Mays Clinic, with hours of being poked and prodded and having to drink chemicals, having chemicals injected into my veins and then having a vein blown out when the contrast was quickly shot into my liver during the CT scan.

Dr. C was engaging and smart, a former New Mexican, and handsome, just like Doris said. He sat down, smiled, and admired my lucky Zuni stone fetish necklace. We talked about green chile and Santa Fe, and then he said the magic words: "I've been through your records and scans. You're ready for surgery," followed with the other magic words: "With this surgery and some cleanup chemo, your chances of five-year survival are 65 percent. At least that's how it goes with my patients."

That was the best news I've heard since last November. There were tears from all of us.

There was more talk and lots of explaining by Dr. C, my new best friend. No, the surgery can't be done laparoscopically, and yes, my bikini days are probably over, but I suspected that a couple of years ago. There were lots of instructions, with Johanna taking fast notes. Dr. C said, "Your liver will regenerate itself, but you have to eat lots of protein. Your diet should be about seventy percent protein after surgery, and you'll have to give up the wine until after you heal." I was happy to agree to that. Wine only tastes good on my off week anyway.

We had lots of questions for him based on our own research. It was comforting that he remembered Doris, whose colon and liver he had sliced open more than a decade ago. He wanted to know about the ranch and about Ray and all the kids. He felt like a hometown guy to me.

I liked him a lot, and I liked his staff. With the news he gave us, there wasn't anything not to like. He scheduled me to be in Houston on March 27 for a pre-op visit and then surgery the following day. The plan was for two to three days in surgical ICU, another five or six days in the hospital, and then maybe another week in Houston recovering in a hotel room. Then I'd have a final visit with him and two months of recovering at home.

We were euphoric heading to the airport. I still have cancer, but you take the good news wherever you can find it. It would have been better only if he had said he wanted to schedule me for next week. Avastin, which is my trial drug, makes for a lot of bleeding (that would explain the daily nosebleeds I've been having) and slow healing, so we now wait five weeks for that to wear off.

The good news is, no more chemo between now and surgery, and then no chemo for the two months that I'm healing. He'll look at my tumor's DNA results, tweak my treatment, and let me know what's recommended after that.

I carried the red notebook with me. *Surgery!, Dr. C, my kids with me, slumber party, No More Chemo.*

No more punching holes in my port and having to carry around a fanny pack with a line into my chest for forty-eight hours, no more bad taste in my mouth, hopefully no more runny noses or headaches or watery eyes for a while. Fewer nosebleeds. Hearing that chemo can stop for a while makes the prospect of surgery not so terrible after all. I understand that after the healing is done, I'll need cleanup chemo, but there really is a light at the end of this tunnel.

I'm ready to be looking back on it more than anything. A bit freaked out by the idea of a big incision and being under and having my entire right and transverse colon removed along with a slice of my liver, but hey, I still have my hair, right? Except for the fact that it's starting to thin. A lot.

Now that I won't have chemo fatigue or those incessant bloody noses, the plan is to get back in good physical shape. Johanna has created a workout schedule for us, with a list of ab-strengthening exercises that I swear I'll follow faithfully. I will be the best surgery patient Dr. C has ever had. I always had to get the highest grade in all my classes in school. Now I plan to be the star patient at MD Anderson.

And maybe we'll get another slumber party, my kids and me. This time, we'll get to include Lesley and my new grandson, who should be on the ground by mid-March. That will make it all worth it.

Chapter 33
Put Me In, Coach

⌁⟶

We are in full-on surgical prep these days. In less than a month, we will be in Houston for my colectomy and liver resection. For now, the chemo is over. I wake with renewed energy and do things like clean out a closet or drawer. I write four blog posts and talk to a couple of clients. I want to come home from surgery with everything in order. I tend to never care much about order and precision and the house being clean, but looking forward to this surgery makes me excited to be alive, makes me want everything to be perfect for my postsurgical, hopefully post-cancerous self when we pull back into the driveway sometime in early April.

Johanna keeps a schedule of workouts and drags me to the Fort Marcy Complex on a daily basis to spend half an hour on the treadmill and alternating days of strength training or ab workouts. It's working. I'm feeling stronger, and really, she's not having to drag me. I go willingly most times. This is for real. Put me in, Coach.

Johanna is still doing coursework online, finishing her final semester at UNM. She has papers due and articles to write and senior projects, which take big blocks of time. After she's done what she needs to do for me, she retires to her room, gets on her Mac, and works. I'm proud and grateful for her, but at the same time, I feel guilty for depriving her of her final semester as an undergrad. She reassures me that this is exactly where she wants to be, but I still feel like it's a shitty way to have to spend your final semester of college. We'll be in Houston for my surgery during her midterms. How exactly will that work?

People are volunteering to go with us. I have a dozen friends and family who are willing to drop whatever they're doing to be with us during my surgery and recovery. I have to say no to some of them, only because it doesn't make sense to have too large a crowd there. And it's not like Houston is just around the corner. It's a fourteen-hour drive from Santa Fe.

Glena and Yvette were the first to call when they heard when I was scheduled.

"I'm a nurse, dammit," Yvette says over the phone. "I'll know exactly how to take care of you."

I'm relieved. Larry credits Yvette with saving him after his colon cancer surgery, and I want her more than anyone else. We have been friends since our grown-up sons were little boys.

Glena will be very helpful. Besides being one of my oldest friends, she's levelheaded and practical and she and Johanna get along well.

Of course, my parents feel like they should be there for the surgery, and there is a bit of a scramble to see who will travel with them. They're capable for a couple their age, but Houston is a morass of bad traffic and one-way streets, and the medical-center complex is exactly what the name says—complex.

My sister, Belinda, and her husband, Andy, end up being the best choices for traveling with Mom and Dad. They lived and worked in Houston for years and know their way around.

So now we have the cast and crew assembled. We just need someone to yell, "Action!"

I'm ready.

CHAPTER 34

You Just Have to Be Pissed Off

~~→

We are two weeks out from surgery when I get the call from Glena.

"Bunny, I have really bad news," she says, and I brace myself. I know her tone of voice. Someone's been in a car accident. Someone's had a heart attack. Someone from our wide circle of friends has died.

"Jerry has stage four prostate cancer."

I'm stunned. My best pal, Yvette, the nurse who is going to come to Houston and be my own personal Nurse Ratched, has been married to Jerry for almost five years. They are a golden couple, my idea of what can happen if you're patient and hope for the best. Yvette has been in two stinking, awful marriages, and then, well into her forties, she met Jerry and fell deeply in love. They have a bloodhound named Festus. Guys who have dogs like Festus shouldn't get cancer.

Jerry's an anesthesiologist in Lubbock. Because of a history of health problems, including a father who died early of colon cancer, Jerry's a health nut. As Yvette says, "He hasn't eaten a single thing he liked since 1985." He works out. He eats lean white meat if he eats meat at all, which is a damn big deal for a guy from West Texas. He's thin as a rail and has never smoked.

He gets scanned on a regular basis for colon cancer. He never drinks too much. He makes the rest of us look like sloths.

I've always thought of myself as the healthiest person in our circle of friends. I've never had a cigarette in my mouth, and I've always gone for a daily walk or a run. Jerry's healthier than me.

But Jerry having stage IV prostate cancer? At fifty-one?

Cancer is so unfair. It's a total bastard. It is so random and without rhyme or reason. I don't get it. There is no discrimination. Why do those of us who feel like we've played by all the rules end up being the sickest? "Who's in charge here?" I want to yell at God.

I immediately text Yvette and tell her not to worry about Houston, but to call me when she has a chance. I think maybe I might be able to dredge up one right thing to say to her.

When we finally talk, she has a hard time explaining what's going on. "He's had a backache for weeks and we thought it was just because he moved some heavy furniture. But finally, I made him go to the doc, and they made him get X-rays. And then a CT scan. Evidently, the cancer we didn't even know was there has now metastasized to his pelvic bones."

Fucking cancer. I am so sick of fucking cancer, and now Yvette can't be in Houston with me because fucking cancer has gotten Jerry. I cry, she cries, and we both say "fucking cancer" aloud three or four times.

"The funny thing is that Jerry has to be at MD Anderson for a consult the day before your surgery. So I'll be there anyway," Yvette says at some point when we've finished cursing God and the universe together. Somehow, I know that God gets it and understands our anger.

We make vague plans to somehow find one another in the medical complex, and I can't help thinking about the irony. I get off the phone. I am truly pissed off at God now. My getting cancer wasn't enough for Yvette to have to deal with right now?

My gut slicing wasn't trauma enough for my crowd of friends to endure this March? You had to give Jerry a totally different form of stage IV cancer? We all had to hear the words "stage IV cancer" once more, less than six months after me?

I email the Wine-Drinking Bible Study girls through my tears and ask them to begin to pray in earnest for Jerry. I also say that I need their prayers as well, that I am in a fury over this new development. I don't get Yvette for surgery, and in addition to worrying about me, she has been completely blindsided by her husband's illness.

Some days, faith just isn't enough. Some days, you just have to be pissed off. Once again, there's nothing I can think to write in the red notebook. I'm too angry.

CHAPTER 35
Dirty Rooms and Recliners

∿➤

Johanna and I are in Houston, getting ready for my pre-surgical consult. It was supposed to be Johanna, Zachary, and me headed to Houston, with Lesley staying at home with Baby Nolan. But Baby Nolan has chosen to delay his arrival. He's now five days overdue. We left Santa Fe almost a week ago, traveling to Logan for one night. Then we drove to Dallas, where we spent three nights, overstaying our welcome, but so certain that we would be helping with the new baby that it never occurred to us that we were arriving early. I wanted three days with my grandson before surgery and instead, he is still *in utero*.

We are staying at a Sleep Inn near the medical center, and it's awful. I'll have to sleep in a recliner for a few days after I'm released from the hospital due to my ab incision. At home, I have a beautiful new electric leather recliner from American Home Furnishings. Here, all I knew was that I had to have a recliner and a kitchenette, and I finally found a place with decent reviews that didn't cost $200 per night. Knowing I might be here nine to fourteen nights required a lot of financial wrangling. But the recliner is included.

It's nasty. Dirty nasty, with dark teal carpet from the '80s that makes me never want to take my shoes off. Are we really going to stay here through my surgery and my hospitalization and the days Dr. C says we need to stick around after surgery? That could be up to two weeks.

It smells like Houston looks, which to me means dark, dank, and moldy. I know it is only March, but it's already wet and sticky. Houston in springtime.

Johanna and I drove here from Dallas in a snarl of traffic that started about 150 miles out, with crowded freeways that made me grip the armrest in fear. Houston traffic is legendary, but until you're in the craziness, you think it's all hype. Not so. It sucks. I'm wrung out by the time Google Maps gets us to Sleep Inn and our room.

We have Dr. C and the anesthesiology consult tomorrow. My parents and Belinda and Andy arrive tomorrow sometime after our meeting with the surgeon. I trust that they will take care of Johanna through the surgery, which is set for Thursday morning. I will be in the hospital for a minimum of five days, Dr. C says, which means I will be released on Monday or Tuesday. Glena is flying in on Saturday afternoon, which is good, since my parents and Belinda and Andy are leaving on Saturday. In the red notebook, I begrudgingly write, *Houston finally, Glena coming, Bendy/Andy, Mom/Dad, Johanna.*

I just don't want Johanna to be alone with me after surgery. She is now the caregiver supreme, but she is still my baby girl.

CHAPTER 36

Wishing for Morphine and Miracles

~~→

I open my eyes in the white-curtained surgical prep area. Johanna is sitting in a chair next to the bed, texting, of course. She spends a lot of time texting these days. I know she's almost always texting someone about me.

"When are they going to take me back?" I ask. We had to be at the hospital at 5:00 a.m. Andy drove the five of us—Mom and Dad, Johanna and me, and Belinda, and dropped us off out front in the cool, foggy Houston morning to go upstairs while he parked the pickup. We found our way to the luxurious family surgical waiting room on the fourth floor, where my dad immediately made three new friends. I knew he'd spend the morning praying some and visiting a lot. That is my dad.

My mom was more reticent than usual. She is on the mend from a bad cold and sinus infection and was almost banned from this trip. You're not allowed to be in the cancer ward if you're sick, so she doubled up on antibiotics and shots and medicine, and now she's looking a bit wan. I suspect that, like me, she didn't sleep a lot last night. I had to drink my GoLytely and clear out my intestines for this procedure, and I was hungry as a bear overnight. And crazy nervous. I don't know what kept her up, but I can guess.

Every consult I had yesterday included me signing a document that said I clearly understood that I could die during the surgery. That'll keep you awake, thinking about how much you don't want to die, how you wish your grandson had arrived on time so you could have held him before today, how you should have mended that one fence with that old friend, how you plan to stay alive to see Jerry get well. And about a thousand other things.

I had strict instructions from Dr. C's nurse: "Nothing by mouth after midnight, including a piece of gum!"

"How about water? Coffee?"

"Absolutely not. When you brush your teeth, pretend you're in a foreign country. Don't swallow, or we'll have to reschedule."

I do not want to reschedule. We have come this far, and I know that if they will ever just get me into surgery, I will be that much closer to cancer-free.

"Johanna," I say again, this time a little louder than the whisper I used before. "When are they going to take me back?"

She looks up in surprise. Her eyes are slightly red-rimmed, I'm supposing from anxiety and the nights of sleeping on Zach and Lesley's couch before we drove to Houston to check into our moldy hotel.

"Mom! You're awake."

"Yes. Just wondering when we'll get to go back."

The nurse comes through the panels. "Breathe!" she says very sternly. "You have to breathe more deeply."

"Mom, you've already been back. It's over."

I don't get it. I was here, in this very place, just a minute ago. Dr. C's assistant surgeon came in and introduced himself and talked about the procedure, going over the risks once more. Then there was the head of the anesthesiology team, and then the respiratory monitor team leader. They were, all three of them, amazingly beautiful young men. I told Johanna it was like MD Anderson hired only soap-opera-pretty people for the roles of medical staff. My nurse looks like a supermodel.

"Really?" I ask, and gingerly touch my stomach. There is no dressing and no pain.

"Yes, it's all done."

"Breathe deeply, Ms. Terry," the nurse says sharply. "You're not getting enough oxygen."

I breathe deeply. Something is beeping around my ear, and I can tell it's an alarm of sorts. But I am wide awake. I cannot have missed every part of the surgery, can I?

"How did I not know I went back? Wasn't I awake when they wheeled me in?"

Turns out, I was awake. But then I had the miracle drug, Propofol, that made me forget every part of the prep, the insertion of the epidural into my spine—everything. The epidural was discussed in my anesthesia consult. It's supposed to help with the pain for the first forty-eight hours. Right now, I'm floating, and there's no pain at all. I'm liking this.

Johanna and the nurse are adamant that I must breathe more deeply. Evidently, another thing the epidural does is make my lungs less efficient. I have lazy lungs. And I'm swimming out from under anesthesia.

"How long was I gone?" I ask.

"About two and a half hours," Johanna says.

I drift in and out, and the nurse sharply tells me to breathe more deeply, that I can't go up to my room until my oxygen levels go up. I think I'm breathing deeply, but obviously she's not happy with me.

Johanna goes out, and my mom comes in. She looks tired and unwell. I don't know it now, but she will go home from this trip and end up horribly ill, in the hospital for almost two weeks with *C. diff*, which is an infection due to the antibiotics killing all the good flora in her own colon. We will nearly lose her. I'll be quarantined from her for a month. But we don't know this now. All we know right now is that I made it through surgery. We're on the other side and relieved.

I'm eventually moved to the surgical ICU ward. Larry told me about this part, that the morphine drip has the potential to make me crazy, that the pain will be brutal, that the nurses will boss me into walking almost immediately. It is just after noon. My family surrounds me, moving about from chair to chair, out into the hall for coffee, downstairs for food. I hear that the cafeteria is beautiful and the food delicious. My dad congratulates me on finding the fanciest hospital in the world for my surgery. There are no rules about when they can be in the room with me, and I guess I sleep for a few hours.

When I wake and try to roll over onto my side, the pain in my abdomen is searing. It is unbearable. The nurse comes in to check my incision. This will happen over and over and over. I have a straight cut from below my belly button to about nine inches above it. It is angry and red, but very clean, and looks like it's superglued together and stapled. Thankfully, I didn't have to have drain tubes. I have twenty-seven staples holding my gut together. And it hurts like a sonofabitch. I have the morphine drip, but the pain doesn't seem to ease when I punch it.

They're going to make me get up and walk feeling like this? I don't think so, although I've planned for weeks to be the model patient.

Dr. C comes to see me late in the day. He takes my hand and says, "How's my star patient?"

I smile. I always worked to be the teacher's pet, and maybe that's what I am with Dr. C. "You tell me."

"It was exactly how I thought it would be. I got it all, including a couple of hot spots close to your existing tumor. I took out twelve lymph nodes. And, like we discussed, I took out your gallbladder as well. It had some scar tissue and didn't look good. You don't want anyone to have to go in there again, do you?"

"Tell me about the liver," I say. I have such a crush on Dr. C. I just want to keep him talking.

"Only five percent had to be resected. Pretty good, I'd say."

I ask about the Propofol. "Did I do anything embarrassing while I was awake that I don't remember?" I'm certain that I probably flirted with him and all the handsome assistants I met earlier.

He laughs. "People do and say some very funny things when they're under like that. But don't worry. We won't tell anyone."

So, yeah, I probably offered some sort of sexual favors to my surgeon.

"And now we're going to get you up and have you start walking," he says.

I'm on a liquid diet for a couple of days while the staples holding my colon together heal enough for food to pass through. It doesn't matter. I'm not hungry, and I don't want to walk around. I want to go to sleep and wake up totally healed and pain-free.

Instead, the nurse comes in after he leaves and tells me it's time. I have to get up and move about. I've just had my gut cut open this morning, and already I'm getting up. Johanna and my mom and Belinda are there. My dad has left the room. I think he's having a hard time with my pain levels. I try not to whine, and the nurse instructs me on the best way to get out of bed. I remember this from Larry's instructions.

"Turn on your right side and use your elbow for support. Try not to use your core muscles to raise yourself off the bed. Lean on your right elbow and push yourself up with your left fist flat on the bed. We'll be here to help you."

The pain is savage, breathtaking, awful. How can I move when I feel like this? I somehow get myself sitting up on the side of the bed, Johanna on one side and the nurse on the other. I am shaking and sweating from the effort. I cry without knowing I'm crying.

"Okay, now we're going to stand. Very slowly."

My nurse is a sweet, friendly girl from South Houston. I know this because my parents have already made her their best friend. She will be my day-shift nurse for the next two days, and then she'll go home to celebrate Easter weekend with her family. I will eventually love her, but right now I despise her.

On the first try, when I raise myself, with Johanna on one side, Belinda on the other, and the nurse in front of me, my blood pressure shoots out of control, and I cry some more.

"Sugar, you lie back down for half an hour. We're going to try this again after your blood pressure calms down."

I complete the unbearable task of lying back down, crying the entire time. I can't stand this pain, yet all the medical personnel assure me it's better than it would be without the epidural. We wait. I dread her return. I hit the morphine button.

Finally, once again and with help, I stand. I shuffle. I cry, tears showing up even though I'm unaware of how they got there. I bend over to protect my screaming gut. I'm sure the tiniest wrong move will send my guts spilling out onto the sparklingly clean floor. Johanna walks on one side, and Belinda walks on the other. I make it down one side of the nurse's station before I feel like I'm going to pass out.

"Okay. Back to bed with you," my nurse says.

I will do this over and over for the next two days, thinking that I'm going to be in ICU for at least four or five days. But at the end of the second day, Dr. C's assistant will come in and say I'm being moved out of ICU. "You're doing great," he'll say, and I'll think, *Uh, yeah, except for my incision hurting like hell every time I roll over. Every time I breathe.*

I learn tricks. After the epidural is removed, I'll ask for hydrocodone on a regular basis, and I'll know I need to let at least two crackers dissolve in my mouth before each dose. In a few days, I'll have graduated from a liquid diet to a very soft diet, so I'll eat broth and yogurt until I'm sick to death of it.

I have my mom and dad and Belinda in my room almost continually through Friday and Saturday, along with Johanna, of course. We visit, Johanna posts about my progress on Facebook, and people comment and call. I truly am a rock star for at least two days, but I don't have the energy to follow along. I don't write in the red notebook. I do nothing other than punch the morphine button and try to walk.

My parents and sister are headed home on Saturday, and Glena is flying in to be Johanna's companion and helper with me. At one point, we talked about not needing help, but it's clear now that I'm too much of an invalid. I'd wear Johanna out if she were all alone.

We are worn out together. We're going to need help.

CHAPTER 37

Pooping the Bed on Easter Sunday

~~→

It is Easter Sunday. I wish I was at Christ Church to celebrate. I am out of ICU, where I spent only two days. Instead of being in a new dress at church, I'm naked in the shower with Glena and Johanna helping me wash my hair. In fact, they're helping me stand. This is an indignity I could have skipped, but I'm too weak and my gut hurts too badly to do it any other way. Glena, I don't mind so much. We have traveled together for years and shared hotel rooms and slept naked together, just because we're girls who sleep naked. She's seen my body in a dozen incarnations. This one is not so pretty.

But Johanna shouldn't have to wash her naked mother's hair. She shouldn't have to know that I pooped the bed this morning. The news of me pooping in the bed is what has the nurses calling my docs, who are now saying that maybe I can go home to my moldy hotel room this afternoon. Pooping after your colon has been stapled together is evidently the biggest damn deal of the day. This is how I'm celebrating the Resurrection this year. I so wish I were in Santa Fe celebrating Easter in a new dress rather than here.

Dr. C's team has come by several times in the past two days. They're cheerful and charming, still seeming like a team of actors from a soap opera. They all want to check my incision, and they comment on how good it looks.

"You're doing so well," they all say in one form or another. I'm sure they're right, but what I know is that if I could choose, I would go through childbirth all over again rather than experience this ab pain. I take the maximum allowed pain meds and worry that I'll get addicted or see visions. Then I worry that I won't stay ahead of the pain. They removed the epidural in the middle of the night last night, along with the catheter. The nurse said I had to be able to urinate in at least two hours, or they would reinsert the catheter. I was immediately on it.

"Get me up. I can urinate right now."

She laughed. "No, it will take a while for the epidural to wear off and for you to feel the urge. Just ring me when you need to get up and go."

It took me a lot of concentration and four glasses of water, but I figured out a way to urinate in two hours.

Johanna or Glena could spend the night with me here, but the care is so good that I've sent them home every night. This is like being in a luxury hotel, except they'll clean the bed if you poop in it. The people who deliver the food are dressed in formal black jackets, looking like a catering service for a benefit dinner. And the food appears to be good, although I've just been a broth eater for the past couple of days. I think longingly of chile rellenos or fried chicken or that delicious green chile queso from Junction in Santa Fe, but I know I'll have to wait a couple of weeks for those meals. Maybe longer.

For now, I'm getting my hair washed, which is its own luxury. Glena finishes with the rinsing. At least the very large bathroom in this private room is all tile and the shower is open so that water runs into a drain in the floor. There is room for all three of us, and I'm the only one getting wet. Johanna turns off the water, and they very gently pat me dry. My belly has a long, ugly gash with all those staples; I look like Frankenstein. Standing this long makes me lightheaded.

But I like finally being clean. I haven't had a shower since early Thursday morning before surgery. Glena combs my hair and gets out the blow dryer. She knows I want to look presentable for the soap-opera doctors. And anyone else I might run into.

The thought that I might be able to go "home" today is crazy. The plan in the first meeting with Dr. C was that I would probably spend a minimum of two to three days in ICU and another three to five days in a surgical ward. We are currently three days after surgery, and I could be going home. I'm apprehensive but ready to get some actual rest. There is a recliner waiting in my moldy hotel room, and I'm looking forward to getting into it and watching movies with Johanna and Glena. My niece, Kyla, is going to fly down to spend a night with us as well. It will almost be like a slumber party. With painkillers.

Meanwhile, back in Dallas, there is still no Baby Nolan. He is now officially ten days late, and we are either texting Zachary on an hourly basis to see if there are contractions, or he texts us to see how I'm doing. I can't wait to get out of Houston and head to Dallas. I want to hold my grandson.

Except that I can't lift anything heavier than a gallon of milk. He'd better not be a big baby.

I haven't written in the red notebook for several days. I'm not sure I know where it is. But I'm still grateful for a lot of things.

CHAPTER 38
Puking in the Trash Can

∿➤

I am sprung from the hospital. Seventy-nine hours ago, we were riding in Andy's pickup from the hotel to the hospital. Now I'm waiting for the orderly to come with a wheelchair to take me down to the first floor. Johanna has gone to the parking garage to retrieve my car. Glena waits here with me. We talk about Yvette's Jerry and how odd it is that he and I are the ones with cancer. We're the nonsmokers. Jerry is the health nut. How did this happen? What the hell is going on? And how did we both end up being stage IV?

Yvette came by my hotel to say hello the day before my surgery. Jerry and his brother waited in the car in the hotel parking lot while she and I sat on a bench, arms around each other, wondering how the hell we ended up in this situation. After all the nights spent dancing with cowboys, music festivals, and shopping together, we were sitting outside a seedy hotel, steps away from MD Anderson.

"Jerry says this is what will kill him," she says, tears in her eyes, "but I told him he had to get his ass down here to have an expert tell me that."

I tell her about the Martin prayer, how the only thing they can do is the thing right in front of them. "You'll make yourself crazy if you think ahead even a day."

"Does that mean you're not thinking about your surgery?"

She knows better. "Is it true that they take my colon out, put it on a table, and work on it?" I ask her. She's a nurse. I expect her to know everything.

"Who cares what they do when you're under? They'll play some great music and do what they're supposed to do. I wish I could be here to take care of you after."

"Take care of Jerry, Love," I say, and I hug her. She lingers, her arms around me, squeezing. She tells me later that she got in the car and Jerry's brother said, "You New Mexico women. Bunny looks great, and you're sitting out there smiling and laughing and chatting like it's any other day in the world. That's some kind of brave."

I wish I had known he said that before the surgery. I didn't feel "some kind of brave." Resigned, perhaps. Tired of having cancer. Tired of not having the life I had planned on.

The news for Jerry was that they'll start immediate immunotherapy. At least that's what I understand from Glena. He's now at the top of my prayer list. I've moved myself from that spot.

I've now performed all the tricks I needed to in order to be discharged. I've eaten cream of wheat for breakfast and tried to stomach a bit of chicken broth and crackers for lunch, and even had one bite of baked chicken. My first meal after surgery. My Easter dinner.

Glena gathers up the last bag of my belongings. I hoist my aching gut and my slow self into the wheelchair with the help of Glena and the orderly. Everything hurts, including my head, but I am determined to get to the curb, to the car. This wheelchair is more like a cart, with room on the back for my bag and the vases of flowers I've received from the Wine-Drinking Bible Study girls, from Jeanne and Pharr, from the Baptist Church in Logan, and an Easter basket from Lesley's mom Carol.

As we leave, I wave to the staff around the nurse's station. They've held my life in their hands, and they've treated me well. This has been like having a resort weekend in a clean, attractive space, but with a long line of Frankenstein staples holding my stomach together. I feel like the wrong move will rip me open, so I carry myself like a newborn child. *I'm becoming a bit of a whiner,* I think.

The orderly works on keeping the bumping to a minimum. We go around corners in the rabbit warren of hallways, moving toward the elevator. The odd lunch, my pain, my subsequent pain meds, and the smell of the flowers behind my head are slowly building up in my goofy gut, and I know I'm going to be sick. I look at Glena in a panic.

"What?" she asks, a bit breathlessly, and I nod toward the flowers. "What do you want me to do?"

"Get rid of them," I say through clenched teeth, "and find me something to throw up in."

I don't want to throw up because I'm fearful of what it will do to my fragile stomach incision. But I don't get to choose. In a fog, Glena grabs a trash can we're passing, holds it under my chin, and I puke and puke and puke some more. And then I cry.

CHAPTER 39

That was Nothing

∿➤

We make it out of the hospital and into the car. Johanna is wide-eyed in the driveway of the hospital, seeing me so pale and shaken, and Glena shakes her head. "Let's just get her home," she says, and they do.

Except that home is a moldy smelling room in a "suite" at our hotel. As we had expected, I cannot lie flat because my incision is so tight and painful, so they've turned the recliner into a bed for me. I slide into it, not very gracefully, with their help and then I ask for my hydrocodone.

Here is where we'll stay for the next six days. I can't get up on my own for the first day or two. That means that I wake either Johanna or Glena to go to the bathroom in the middle of the night. The toilet extender is a lifesaver. Thank you, Larry and Shelley, for insisting that I get one. This one is a gift from Belinda and Andy. Who knew I would be so grateful for a new toilet seat? If I could find the red notebook, I'd write it in there.

I can hardly sit down to pee. I never knew I used my ab muscles for so many things, like sitting on the toilet. And bowel movements are their own adventure. Once I'm done, we have to examine everything for fresh blood and alert the nurse on call if there's an issue.

We watch a lot of television. Every couple of hours, Johanna makes me get up and walk the halls of our moldy hotel, her and Glena on either side of me as I shuffle toward the lobby, hunched over my sore stomach muscles. I would be a spectacle anywhere else, but here, I am just one more patient getting over one more procedure. Hotels near the medical center are filled with people like me. I am nothing special.

Here's the good news. On Sunday afternoon, after the puking in the hospital hallway, after the grueling ride back to the hotel, after the difficult walk from the car to the room, after the grits for dinner, Zachary called and said Nolan was officially on the way. He called again later in the evening and said Nolan was a 9-pound, 11-ounce, C-section baby who had finally arrived. I am happy. I can lift ten pounds, or at least hold it in my lap. That means that Baby Nolan made it in just under the wire. We admire cellphone photos and post on Facebook. Baby Nolan and I have both made it. Happy Easter to all of us.

By Tuesday night, we are all a little sick of each other and our ugly room. Glena and Johanna make noises about going out to find food. I send them off. I am fine by myself, and we are all experiencing severe cabin fever. We've had a call from Kyla, and she'll be here tomorrow to give everyone a break. Glena will go home.

I am finally alone while my caregivers go to Rice Village to have a break from me. I lean my head back against my pillow on the recliner and allow myself to cry silently, tears running down into my ears. I am so tired, so sick of pain meds and the shuffling down the halls and the smell of Houston in general. I also look like shit, pale and wan with ugly hair, whatever hair I still have.

I am so scared that I'll open up my surgical wound, that Johanna will never want to spend another minute with me after this, that I'll never go on another date, that my scar will never look okay, that I'll never be naked in the presence of another human again. I do not know how this got to be my life. I know I am supposed to be grateful, that I should read the Facebook posts and the cards and the emails from all over the country, the ones that say people are praying for me and that they're proud of me and that they find me an inspiration.

I think about a year ago at this time, the months after Last Boyfriend dumped me after three years for someone twenty years younger, about my whining and moaning and crying all the time. It felt so monumental at the time, like something I would never get over. Now, with my gut stapled together and my possible cancer-free status in front of me, I wonder who that whiner was. How did I allow myself to be the person who would settle for that life with him? What was I thinking?

That was nothing. This is something.

CHAPTER 40
Chemo Despair

∿➤

Tomorrow is chemo again. Treatment number seven. Since December, I've had six treatments, a six-week break, surgery to remove all my tumors and twelve lymph nodes, and then a more-than-six-week recovery period. It's now May. My yard is greening up, and I'm feeling some energy after my surgery recovery. But I have to go back for more chemo. I don't even try to hold the tears at bay. Again? Really?

Today is Monday. I just dropped off my kids at the airport in Albuquerque and drove back to Santa Fe alone. Zachary, Lesley, and Baby Nolan leave for Dallas at 2:00 p.m., and Johanna leaves for Kansas to spend a week with her dad's family, and to attend a cousin's graduation, right after that.

I dreaded the drop-off. I was exhausted last night thinking about being all alone in this house that's been filled with laughter and baby noises, Zach and Johanna teasing each other, and all of us watching a marathon of season two of *Game of Thrones*. While Baby Nolan cooed on the couch or in my lap, we had conversations about the future. We just completed Johanna's UNM graduation weekend, me prouder than I could say that she did so well and ended up with a 3.9 GPA after having to take care of me and endure this cancer bullshit for the past six months.

At the party at my sweet Albuquerque friend Jolynn's house following the graduation ceremony, I made a toast, saying, "Back in November when I was diagnosed, there were two things that made me determined to get well: Nolan's birth and Johanna's graduation from college. I was sure that if I could get to those two events, I could get to cancer-free. And here we are. Johanna has accomplished more in her final semester of school than any of you can imagine…" and then I choked up, and someone else had to take over.

Six months. I was diagnosed on November 10, 2012, and Johanna graduated on May 10, 2013. We didn't talk about this being any sort of milestone. I only realized the coincidence of the dates after the event. At the moment that Dr. L used the words, "stage IV colon cancer," all I could think about was Johanna's graduation and the baby being born in March. "Get me there," I prayed, while Dr. L talked about tumor markers, chemotherapy, and possible surgeries. "Get me to March and May."

So here I am, tumor-free, but still forced by modern medical science to go through more treatments. At my Houston follow-up with Dr. C eight days after surgery, he said, "I can't tell you what to do, but the protocol is for you to have a series of cleanup chemo treatments. Talk to your oncologist about it. He wants you to stay well." He had been happy with the results of the surgery and my quick recovery. "Come back to see me in August," were his instructions.

Mari Anne will pick me up this morning and take me to chemo, staying for a few hours until Jennifer can take her place and drive me home. Johanna is getting a break from this round. Surely by now, I can handle this alone. I have happily (at least in her presence) let her go to Kansas.

When I began treatments back in December, I was frightened. There were so many unknown factors, and the thought of being hooked up and being on the infusion pump after I left the chemo suite was daunting. I didn't know how the pump would work, or feel, or how I would do being hooked up to something while I slept or bathed or dressed.

Now I'm just tired of the process. I am sick to death of cancer treatments. I want to be done. I want my life back. I want to move on and spend my time planning my future instead of waiting two weeks for another treatment.

Dr. L has insisted on my doing a minimum of six more treatments. I've already made my mind up that I'm refusing six treatments and that I'll do only four. *Get me through June,* I'm thinking, *and I'll be done with these treatments, and I'll go to Houston to see Dr. C in August.* Then, if Dr. C sees something that he thinks warrants more treatments, I'll do the remaining two. But I know I won't need them.

I will go and have this treatment and the next and the next. I will trudge along this path for a bit longer. In the red notebook, I write, *Johanna's graduation, Nolan and Zach and Lesley, everyone I love healthy.* I do not write *More chemo.*

CHAPTER 41

Start from Here

∿→

Start from here. Start from here. Start from here. I am trying to make that my mantra these days. This past week has been ugly. I thought the ugly part of my life was over. But I started chemo again. I've treated myself with kid gloves and allowed myself to wallow in self-pity while refusing to do anything productive. You would think that after being diagnosed in November, starting chemo in December, having surgery to remove all my tumors in March, and recovering for weeks, during which I was tumor-free, I'd be more than happy to begin chemo again to get this thing wrapped up and done.

Instead, I've been unhappy and angry and sad, on the verge of tears all week. Going back to that chemo suite, getting my port flushed, and being on the infusion pump for forty-eight hours feels like the worst sentence in the world. It feels like defeat. And the ensuing fatigue and headaches and sick stomach have been the worst — maybe not because they really were the worst, but because I felt so sorry for myself for having to go through this process again. Good grief, I am a baby about this.

Jeanne says to give myself a break, that when I began chemo last time, I was not a postsurgical patient and therefore probably felt better physically and not so washed out. But I feel as if I've been giving myself a break for a long time now.

I need to be more productive, I need to work harder, I need to be better organized, I need to get more clients, work harder, et cetera, et cetera, et cetera. I worry about money all the time, not because I don't have any savings left from the sale of my house, but because at the rate I'm going, I will be broke by November or December. And that's multiplied by the fact that I haven't been doing much work for my online clients while treating myself with such care and being a total sloth.

But as Jeanne says, maybe I need to give myself a break. There is the problem of chemo brain, which is very real. While this chemo makes my gut ache and I'm exhausted, my brain is foggy all the time. Jeanne says this is the combo of the chemo and the anesthesia still in my system from the surgery. I'm still on Ambien to sleep, which doesn't help.

Start from here, start from here, start from here. I promise that I will start my life from here, from this place where I am mostly healthy, mostly sane, working on being more productive and creative. I am just so tired.

Perhaps the chemo is more brutal now because there is no cancer to treat. I read somewhere that the people who get hooked on prescription drugs are the ones who don't need them and that the drugs have a stronger effect when they have no pain to relieve. Maybe that's how chemo is. Now that there is no big fat chubby tumor to shrink, the chemicals are eating away at my good health. And my good health is not such great health right now, having survived the initial onslaught of six treatments and all that anesthesia and those drugs and the surgery itself. I don't feel strong in any way.

After the surgery, I asked Dr. C if I was cancer-free. "Well, technically, your tumors are gone, along with the lymph nodes that were affected. Let's talk about this again in August when you come back."

Today I have one chemo treatment down, three to go. Dr. L wants me to have six treatments. I want four. After months of doing whatever the medical community suggested, I am suddenly stubborn.

I have nothing to write in the red notebook. I don't feel grateful. I feel miserable. But I still get it out and write *Jeanne letting me whine, my kids healthy, a photo of Baby Nolan on my phone, clean sheets, eleven days to the next treatment.* It's an exercise I'd like to leave out of my life and yet it does remind me that I can make it another day. *Blinders on.*

CHAPTER 42

Is the Cure Killing Me?

∿➤

A week ago was my absolute last chemo treatment unless they find a recurrence. June 23, 2013. A date I will never forget.

I should be celebrating. But the postsurgical chemo continues to wrack my gut. I search for foods that won't irritate me, but I haven't been successful with anything yet.

Since they removed the pump last Wednesday, my gut has been working overtime, and I have spent hours in the bathroom producing prodigious amounts of shit (I'm past calling it poop. That's a toddler word. The stuff I'm making is not something a toddler would create). I am so ready for it to end. "What's the reason?" I asked Jeanne yesterday while we were sitting under the trees at La Casa Sena, having our Santa Fe version of a coffee break. She ordered a vegetable plate to go with our delicious Marble Brewery Stouts. It arrived with some pita bread and hummus. I eyed both the beer and the hummus warily.

"Jeanne," I said, "Why do you think I'm having such a tough time with my gut? And why am I producing so damn much waste? My doctor doesn't seem to be worried at all."

Her theory is that this means the chemo is working overtime. Its job is to attack growing cells, which are in my stomach lining, my nose, my mouth, my eyes. My stomach lining is having an especially difficult time of it, metabolizing everything I eat into an immediate trip to the bathroom. For the first time in my life, I found myself in the aisle at Smith's looking for Preparation H. I was so relieved when I located it.

Dr. L says this cancer started with a polyp ten years ago. Surprisingly I never had an issue with my bowel habits. *Oh, me?* I'd think. *You can set your watch by when I go to the bathroom. Once in the morning after my cup of coffee, once in the afternoon at about 2:15. No issues. I've never had any issues. Right as rain.*

One would think that colon cancer would give you issues with your bowels while it's growing, not after everything's been removed. The other disturbing fact is that I never had a single symptom other than a side ache one Saturday in October, about a month before my diagnosis, something that felt like I had run a mile just a bit too fast. And the lightheaded feeling that everyone attributed to my hormones. If you're a fifty-one-year-old woman, "It's your hormones, dear," is the answer to everything. We know now that my colon wall was bleeding, the blood slowly seeping into my abdomen.

Other than that, no symptoms. Nothing that required a doctor visit. Certainly nothing that seemed like it could kill me. What would have happened if I had waited for the pain to get worse on that November afternoon? Would I have had an emergency surgery that would have delayed my treatment, lessening my chances of survival on this end?

Now I wonder if the chemo is killing me instead. Friends tell me about how they either heard a doctor in a cancer clinic or someone on a talk show say that in ten years, we'll look back on chemo as the most barbaric thing we did to sick people. Yvette's Jerry continues to fight his stage IV prostate cancer. When she and I talk, we do what I suppose other people did with me: speak to one another in hushed tones, cry a bit, and generally put him on the disabled list until we know what sort of treatment they might continue to prescribe.

He's been put on a trial immuno-suppressant therapy. Some hormones, some melatonin treatment, but something that in less than four monthly treatments has his PSA at a manageable level. The metastases in his bones appears to have gone away. His oncologist, a young woman from Spain, says, "No, there will be no chemo for my patients because chemo is crazy, it causes more long-term bad effects than the actual cancer itself, it eats your bone density, creates secondary cancers, and increases your chance of congestive heart failure!"

I'm crazier than ever these days. If the cancer doesn't kill me, the after effects of the chemo could. Or all those CT scans I've had in the past year. That would so piss me off.

At the disconnect a week ago, the nurses were sweet, and everyone, including Steven, the soothing pharmacist, came by and told me how happy they were for me. The nurses had me choose a surprise from a basket, and it was a flat, white stone with the word "Serenity" on it. "That's perfect for you, Bunny," Jan the Nurse said. "You never sit still, and you're never totally quiet when you're here."

I hear that elsewhere they ring a bell when you're done with chemo. It's a nice touch, but perhaps hard on the folks who are nowhere close to the end of their treatments or to having a bell rung for them. I wish I were more excited about the end of this. I wish I felt better.

I know how chemo works. I know the first few days after a treatment are always the most rugged, and I know the improvement on the days after that is exponential, that I will feel better and better and better until I am my old bundle of energy and my brain starts working again.

To distract myself, I've considered dating again. I get on OkCupid to see what happens. I open my old profile and almost immediately have three messages. I respond to those, and now I have more.

I like the online conversation but not the insistent messages suggesting a meet and greet. What would we do? What would we say? I have dated almost every type of guy in the world, it seems, and I have no idea how to begin again, especially with my story of cancer lurking behind every conversation. I don't want cancer to define me, but right now that's my truth. And I have this scary scar. Who would ever be interested in me, in the in-person me?

I panic, and immediately hide my photos, closing my profile the next day after I read yet another email from a seemingly interested guy. I can't do this craziness right now.

In the red notebook I write THE END OF CHEMO. That will have to be what I'm most grateful this week. It feels like the only thing.

CHAPTER 43

Dancing with My Daughter

∿➤

Two weeks out from my last chemo treatment. Did I make the right choice to cut the chemo short? Should I have had those last two treatments? There's so much conflicting information out there. Dr. L was disappointed when I told him I didn't plan to complete the protocol, that I'm cancer-free, and that I agreed to four treatments after surgery, not six. Could he give me a compelling reason that six is better than four? He said that patients at my stage do six treatments after surgery because it's the protocol, whether you're an eighty-year-old with diabetes or a twenty-seven-year-old in perfect health. He added that I'm unique in that I am now basically cancer-free, and so few of his stage IV patients are cancer-free at this point. I've done my research. I'm feeling stronger every day, and I can't go back for more. I just can't.

There is Dr. L's concern. Then there is the information that says we will decide in a few years that chemo was barbaric, that new autoimmune treatments are the best method, and that chemo causes secondary cancers, early onset of dementia, and porous bones leading to osteoporosis. And there is Sarah, sweet, sarcastic Sarah, who didn't have a surgery like mine, who still has spots on her liver, and who would have been on chemo another year or two or three if Dr. L had his way. She has taken her liver spots to Denver to a specialist who has implanted radioactive beads in her liver to maybe kill the cancer. She tells me not to do more chemo, that these guys at this clinic are crazy, that they would have you on maintenance chemo for years.

There is the internet that says it doesn't matter because I'm basically fucked. The statistics say that only 20 percent of all stage IV patients with colon cancer make it five years. Or sometimes, the number is 2 percent from an alternative cancer center in Phoenix that's trying to get you in for a regimen of something else involving an iridologist and coffee colonics. Two percent is a bit of a bitch to think about, so instead I think of my surgeon, Dr. C, saying on our first visit that the people who have the treatment that I did and then come to him for surgery have better than a 65 percent chance of long-term survival.

I try to hold all these numbers and percentages in my head and then I realize that it doesn't matter. First, my brain no longer works with numbers, and second, if I survive, I'm in the smaller percentage of Dr. L's numbers, the higher percentage of Dr. C's numbers. Maybe.

I apply Mederma skincare cream to my surgical scar every night. I go to Fort Marcy to get on the treadmill every other day, at least. I work as much as possible; I'm back to writing blogs on a daily basis and managing seven social media accounts. The checks from my clients are starting to get bigger. I juice at least one meal a day, and although I'm pretty sure my head should be full of gratitude and working harder and trying to get myself back to incredibly healthy, all I seem to be thinking about is the impossibility of dating.

I'm pretty sure I'm expected to say something about death or how I can help others now that I'm out of the woods, but honestly, I mostly think about dating. With my thousands of friends and my multitude of family, I'm still so lonely. And my friends seem to be bored with me. I'm bored with myself. To distract myself, I think about dating.

I consider reopening the OkCupid profile and posting the Halloween picture, wondering how I think I can now pull off having even a short cup of coffee with guys from OkCupid who might think that the girl in the blue dress is going to show up. I don't look like that anymore. I'm puffy from the steroids. My hair is dry and thin.

And here's the kicker: I don't really want to meet anyone. I just want the *idea* of someone right now. I want to dip my toe in the possibility of someday meeting someone who might be capable of dancing me around the kitchen late some night.

Instead, I take a shower, and Johanna and I head downtown to drink a beer at Marble Brewery, overlooking the plaza while we wait for Alex Maryol to take the stage at the bandstand. July in Santa Fe is a gift, even when you're as morose as I am these days.

"I'm trying to decide whether I want to start dating again or not," I tell her.

"Ugh," she says, "I hate dating. But I love attention."

"That's it! That's what I want."

"Well, there's nothing wrong with letting someone hang around every once in a while," she tells me. "But I don't want to date anyone. I just want someone to be paying attention."

"Right. I know that if I had a man in my life, we'd have him here with us right now. We'd accommodate him instead of having this conversation. And he'd want to do something different from what we're doing, and I'd have to think about when he was coming over, and we'd immediately start doing crap we don't want to do. Am I right?" I ask her.

"I'm telling you, Mom. You don't want to date. You just want the attention."

She is right, as always. I don't want a man cluttering up my life or my household or my head. But I want to know they're out there when I change my mind. When my big ugly gut scar is less frightening. When I look less like a science experiment.

I drag her to the plaza when Alex begins to play. We've been following him for years, since he was seventeen and too young to get into Albuquerque bars without his mom. He's my favorite local guitarist. I stand on the short wall around the obelisk so I can see him better over the heads of the crowd. Johanna is embarrassed. She seems to be the only person in the crowd under fifty. "That's Santa Fe," she says. "Everyone is old except me."

I tell her that now that I'm cancer-free and we've won this battle, she has to dance with me and that it has to be close to the stage. "Oh, Mom," she moans, "now you're going to play the 'I beat cancer' card instead of the straight cancer card?"

But when Alex plays a tune we can dance to, she rolls her eyes and follows me out on the dance floor. I tell her that at the end of her life, she'll wish she danced more. A lot more, even if some of it was with her mother.

A soft rain starts, and we're hungry, so we dance to one more song. I say, "Okay, good. I'm done. Let's go to the Cowgirl and get one of those harvest salads with Chimayó chicken."

CHAPTER 44

Being Alive Is a Good Thing, Right?

∿→

Getting the port out was a bitch. It was just another in the long list of medical procedures I get to check off my list, but this one was painful and left me with a line of stitches and deep bruising on my chest. The bruising is from the doctor having to saw away at the scar tissue that had grown up over the port itself. They shot me up with five or six injections of lidocaine to deaden the area and he started cutting. Every time I felt something sharp, I was to raise my hand, and they'd give me another injection. I had three more after the original round.

I was tense and sweating, and the doc said, "Well, the catheter is out." I thought that meant the end. But no, the device still had to be removed, the small, one-half-inch raised disk into which the nurses poked my chemo needle every time I had treatment. I had been warned that the scar-tissue removal was a bitch. They had my head turned and draped, but I could hear and feel the pressure of him cutting. It felt like sawing to me, which I'm sure it wasn't. It felt crazy, so I tried to transport myself out of that room onto the patio at the Bull of the Woods, where I danced last Friday night with Johanna, Courtney, and Amy to Robert Earl Keen on our trip to celebrate the end of chemo. I thought about floating on a Ute Lake inner tube, cold beer in my hand, my legs tucked up under Angie's tube. I thought about sitting in Zach and Lesley's living room holding Nolan. I thought about every favorite place as quickly as I could.

Now the port is out. Next? Driving to Houston to have more blood drawn, a CT scan, and a consult with a geneticist and my surgeon, Dr. C. I'm sick of medical shit, tired of medical facilities, pokes with needles, and getting stuff put in and stuff taken out.

But I'm alive. That's a good thing, right? I keep waiting to be ecstatic about my recovery. Instead, I am plodding through life. I don't even like myself anymore. I've gone days without writing down a single thing I'm grateful for. I'm a petulant child.

CHAPTER 45

Letting Go

∿➤

It's August. We are in post-cancer mode now. Johanna and I set in Dr. C's office at MD Anderson and wait for him to give us the results of my last CT scan. We are just back from two days on the beach in Galveston, during which we rented beach chairs and an umbrella, carried a cooler filled with a six-pack of Blue Moon down near the water, and sat for hours with our books, sipping beer and occasionally turning to one another to say something that might have been profound had I written it down.

At one point, she said, "Are you scared to see him tomorrow?"

I said, "Maybe. What if the scan shows a tiny little hot spot of something?"

"Yeah," she said, and turned back to her book. I looked out at the waves coming in, that endless water. It would be a nightmare for the cancer to have come back so quickly. It would not mean good things because what I had before was slow growing. I think about a woman I know from Logan, a forty-something mom whose cancer was so advanced and untreatable that she chose not to seek any treatment, and how at her funeral last week, the slide show of her riding horses with her boys and dancing with her husband made us all cry that much more. She was doing stuff like this, hanging with her kids, not knowing she was carrying cancer around only eighteen months ago. Now her youngest son is going to football practice two days a week, and she's not at home at the end of the day to ask him how it went.

I don't know what I would do if the cancer is back. I guess continue to fight it. I don't know what else I could do.

Johanna and I treat ourselves like royalty in Galveston, spending money on whatever restaurant Yelp said had the best fresh oysters, buying beach towels from a souvenir shop, having $16 martinis at the bar in the Hotel Galvez. It feels like an overdue celebration.

Galveston feels bigger than Red River last week with Robert Earl Keen and Courtney and Amy. It feels like us conquering the ugliness that Houston represents for us. We are self-indulgent. My credit card works overtime; I refuse to think about when I will have to pay for all this extravagance.

We deserve it. When the week is over, I'll drive back to Santa Fe alone, and Johanna will stay in her new apartment in Dallas. She'll start grad school at the end of August. I know I'm well and that it's time for her to get on with her life, but she has been my constant companion and my rock—and sometimes, also the irritant that only your children can be. We have watched hours of *Downton Abbey*, crying like we'd lost a member of our family when Sybil died in childbirth, smiling through tears when Mary and Daniel finally made it to one another and kissed in the falling snow on Christmas Eve. She got me addicted to the Kardashians, which Courtney says is one of the worst side effects of my cancer.

But, of course, we didn't only watch television together. She was calm when I wasn't. On the day I cried in the car outside Walgreens about Dr. B (for "bitch") prescribing only seven Ambien when I so desperately needed thirty, she called and threatened to go back to the clinic and kick her ass. When the study coordinator got my scheduling wrong, she figured it out. She made me go for walks after surgery, up and down the halls of our marginal hotel, me bent over like an old lady, holding my stomach. She made me go to movies when I was on the pump and complaining of how I looked like an alien dragging around a fanny pack. "You'll forget you're connected if we go to the movies." She ran interference with anyone who wanted something from me, if only to give me their sympathy.

And now I will have to live alone without her.

The news from Dr. C is good. We sat in his office the day after our last Galveston indulgence, and he came in smiling, hugging us both, and telling us how beautiful we were. He admired my almost-totally-healed scar and said, "You know, your scans were all clean. You're good for another four months." We cried, which is what we seem to do with him.

I will go home and live alone with the good news. I'm still not writing in my red notebook. I'm still unsure what I'm truly grateful for, even though I know that conventional wisdom says I should be happy, happy, happy.

CHAPTER 46
To Whom Much Is Given

～～➤

This is the day of the Christmas Pageant tryouts at Christ Church. I've volunteered to help in whatever way they need me. I'm trying to give back. To whom much is given, much is required, that sort of thing. I'm also dying to get myself back out there in the world, where I'm not moping over my incredibly good fortune. I am sick of being unhappy. I'm bored with my own bad attitude. And I have a really bad attitude.

The Christ Church children's ministry will perform *A Charlie Brown Christmas,* and we'll have rehearsals every Thursday between now and Christmas Eve. I'm going to arrange the rest of my life so that I'm available for every single meeting, audition, rehearsal, set design, whatever is needed. I am going to be excited.

I'm working steadily now, with four new clients and a lot of words to string together in exchange for cash. My brain is foggy, but less so. An old friend says, "You know, Bunny, you might be depressed." I refuse to be still or be depressed. Instead I am determined to hurtle myself headlong into something, anything that will stir up some energy and enthusiasm. I don't even recognize myself in this lethargy.

Last Christmas was such a bust, so full of angst and sorrow and fatigue. I had a chemo treatment on December 22. It wasn't optimal, having a treatment right before Christmas, but then nothing was optimal. It was my second treatment, and the chemo nurse had assured me that the first three wouldn't be horrible, that the side effects would be minimal.

All I remember is that the entire season was tinged with low-level fatigue, along with the constant reminder that I had cancer. I tried not to think forward to this year. I tried to see only the next hurdle in front of me, which felt daunting.

So this Christmas, I get to give something back, all the magic, good feelings, love, and grace that were given to me last year when I thought all I wanted for Christmas was several days in bed. This afternoon, I'll meet with others in the sanctuary. We'll listen to the line reading and watch the thirteen or fourteen kids and teenagers who want to be in *A Charlie Brown Christmas*.

I suspect my job will be herding the baby Woodstocks, the three- and four-year-olds, but that's fine. I need to get myself in the middle of celebrating the season.

Last year, I got it all, but in a fog—chemo, fatigue, Christmas Eve church service, great food, Canyon Road, snowfall, and more. This year, I plan to be awake and alive. I will have had my second surgical follow-up with Dr. C by then, and I will be more reassured than ever that I am getting well. That I *am* well. I will be moving forward.

I'll do Christmas right this year. In addition to the play and Christ Church, I have Baby Nolan to buy for, and Zach and Lesley will be bringing him to Logan for the holiday. This Christmas will be filled with hope and love and grace. I'm sure of it.

I finally write in the red notebook. *Jennifer, Christ Church, Baby Nolan, Christmas coming.* I have no more energy or passion about life than I did yesterday, but it's time to start paying attention to gratitude. Whether I feel it or not.

CHAPTER 47

Why You're Still Single

⌁→

I read an article I see on Facebook titled "22 Reasons You're Still Single." There are some good reasons, such as, "You're a downer," "You treat his friends badly," "You're high maintenance." It's clear this article is written for twenty-somethings: "You're still a party girl." It doesn't address my frequent evenings of watching sports with the old guys at Del Charro, but there are still valid points. Number 6 is "You have trust issues. You can guard your heart and not get hurt again, or you can be vulnerable and experience love. You cannot do both, so you have a choice to make." Yeah, right. And "You're too picky." That could also be true.

I'm wondering if in my case, "You had stage IV cancer, and now you have an ugly 12 inch scar on your gut, and you're afraid of how you'll be perceived" could be a valid reason for me.

I've been on a few dates with one particular guy, and I'm thinking maybe it's okay. I'm not 100% on board, but I am liking it on occasion. He is kind and intelligent, and while he doesn't blow my skirt up, I am taking it very slowly, breathing in and out, wanting to talk to him late at night, trying not to think, think, think. Cancer has made me so tentative about everything that I don't quite know how to act.

When I got the cancer-free news, I expected to be over the top with enthusiasm about getting on with my life. I thought I'd run into the streets shouting. I thought I finally would get to do what I wanted to do when I moved to Santa Fe — reinvent myself into something amazing.

Instead, I very slowly dip my feet into each day and try not to think too much about possibilities. I also try not to think about what any man in his right mind would say if he saw my ugly scar. Whether the cancer will come back. What life is supposed to look like now. What I'll do now that I'm not the center of attention. Mostly, I try not to think.

CHAPTER 48

Today is All You Have to Conquer

~~→

November 10.

I wake at six, thankful I've slept this late given that the recent time change frequently has me up at 4:30 or 5:00. It's Sunday. I'll go to the early service. Tomorrow night, I have the Wine-Drinking Bible Study Group at my house. Gypsy stew, a gluten-free dessert, and wine, of course. I can't wait for them to see my house and the way all my Mexican folk art and tinwork fit in this bright white space with the cobalt blue tile. This may well be the best place I've ever lived, my little Salazar Street house in Santa Fe.

Back in June, when I was in clean-up chemo and needed to find a new place to live because my landlord wanted to sell my Railyard house, I had to move. Sylvia, the Ministry Coordinator at Christ Church, organized a group of twelve men to help me move. Johanna and I packed (helped out by the Christ Church Youth Group on a couple of Wednesday nights) and then on moving day, seven pickups showed up and these men, who were angels in disguise, moved us here. I didn't know then how much I loved this little house. I only knew that my life was surprisingly blessed.

Now I get up, make myself a cup of coffee, and turn on the gas fireplace to warm the front rooms. I get my computer out and, as is part of my morning ritual now, take the computer back to bed. I write for myself in bed. I write for my clients at the desk. The client writing takes up most of each day, but for at least half an hour every day, I give myself a cup of coffee in bed, computer on my lap. One thousand words. That's my contribution to my sanity these days.

When I type the words "November 10" at the top of the page, it hits me. One year. Three hundred sixty-five days. An entire year has gone by since I lay on that table in the gastro lab at St. Vincent's and heard the gastroenterologist say, "Aha! There it is. I've been doing this for seventeen years, and I know cancer when I see it!" She seemed so excited, and in my drugged state, instructed me to look at the screen. There. It. Was. Flashing and pulsing on the screen, angry red. My cancer. There was the meeting in the curtained area with my parents and Johanna, where she told the people I love that I had colon cancer and that my liver was also "involved." And then she said, "I just don't know if this is treatable or not."

That was one year ago today. Today there is no cancer. The angry, pulsing tumor in my colon is gone, my liver is missing a slice off the top right corner, and I am healthier than ever. Or at least healthier than I was a year ago. My gut still doesn't act right when I eat something sweet or spicy. I'm learning as I go what works and what doesn't.

In the past year, I've had it all. Amazing doctors and surgical assistants, fabulous nurses, and then some freaky nurses who scared the bejesus out of me. I've had family and friends gather 'round and cover me up with good wishes and prayers and care. I've learned things I never knew I needed to know, like where to hang out near MD Anderson.

I've had my hometown put together a benefit that raised an astounding amount of money. I've had a grandson born in the midst of it all — Baby Nolan, who gave me the will to get up and get better every morning. I've had a daily phone call with T. J. I've made new friends at the chemo suite. I've walked miles on the treadmill at Fort Marcy.

Mostly, I've had a lot of prayers. And the red notebook to remind me how grateful I am, even when I didn't think I was.

While I was sick, I got letters from small churches in New Mexico, from people I had never met and places I had never been, and the copied body of the letter would say something like, "We just wanted you to know that we are praying for you every day." The letter would be signed by five or six people. I could see them, the Wednesday-night prayer group at the First Baptist Church in Melrose or Hondo or Tatum, with their heads bowed, praying over their lists, my name in the middle. My Facebook page was blown up with promises of prayer. In my mailbox every day, there would be a greeting card from someone saying I was in their prayers. My Aunt Crystell and my Aunt Jackie sent one almost every week. I loved those promises of prayers.

But for me, Martin's prayer on the day of my first oncologist visit, the prayer about having blinders on, that one was the best. When I was facing another chemo treatment, I knew that the next hour was all I had to get through. When I was on my way to Houston for surgery, I was able to break the day down and get through just the one thing in front of me. When the nurses were trying to get me out of bed to walk around the room that first night after surgery, I knew I was only expected to stand. And then to walk five steps. And then to walk to the nurse's station.

I'm eternally grateful for the community of people that sprang up around me in the past twelve months. If there were a way to repay their care and generosity, I'd do it. Instead, here's one thing I can say to them all:

You don't have to conquer your entire life today. You don't have to do anything other than clear the next hurdle that is in front of you. If you can keep blinders on, if you can just handle the next thing with grace and love, fear won't take over your life.

I write in the red notebook, *One year.* That's more than enough for today.

Chapter 49

The Fear Never Goes Away

~~>

December. I'm headed to Houston today for my second follow-up. Eight months since surgery, and Dr. C said he wanted to see me one more time before turning me over to the Santa Fe docs for five years of follow-ups. I'm happy to see him. When a guy saves your life, you fall a little bit in love with him.

I'm in Dallas for a quick visit before Houston. Baby Nolan sleeps in the next room. Zach and Lesley sleep in their bedroom. We were up late last night, playing Catan, which is my least favorite board game in the world, but because they're my kids, I went along. Johanna was here, showing up after her grad school classes to have dinner with us. Now I'm up, far too early for sensible people, but I'm headed to the airport for my Houston flight. I don't want to be late.

I'm making this run to Houston alone. I didn't plan it that way, but that's how it shook out. My sister offered to go along but had to cancel. Johanna has finals this week. I'll fly to Houston alone, go through the scans and blood tests, see Dr. C early tomorrow morning, and fly back to Dallas tomorrow afternoon. I'm not excited.

There's always a lurking fear, always a gut-wrenching thought that the cancer is going to find its way back, that my refusal to do the last two chemo treatments was a death sentence.

I recently stopped by Will's office to see Sarah. I've texted Will a few times to check on things and he's always purposefully vague about how she's doing. "Oh, Bunny, we're just hanging in there," he says, and I gather that things are not fabulous. I feel guilty about being the person who is well. I feel that a lot. When I see Bobby in Logan, whose young wife passed away this summer from cancer a few months past her fortieth birthday, I want to hide somewhere. I know he doesn't resent me for having survived, but I still feel crappy, as if I'm a living rebuke. T. J. calls it "survivor syndrome," and I've never known anything about it before. Whatever it is, I frequently feel guilty that I'm the one who lived.

Since I couldn't get a straight answer from Will, I started saying small prayers about Sarah, asking God to give her some peace and me a chance to check on her. One afternoon on my way home from Target, I stopped in at the construction company office. She was there, looking a bit pale, but otherwise her lovely Sarah self.

The news isn't good. While they were waiting to see how the radioactive seeds planted in her liver were working, spots developed on her lungs. Now she shows me her new port.

"Yeah, so I had to have another fucking port put in," she says, and I know that I'd say exactly the same thing. She's being treated in Albuquerque now and has a scan in the next couple of weeks to see if this new round of chemo is working.

"I told my doctor this is it. No more chemo after this. He says it's the highest-powered stuff available, and it's kicking my ass. If this stuff doesn't work, I'm done," she says.

I don't know it at the time, sitting on the other side of that desk, but Sarah will not survive this new fight. The cancer will be too much, and the Albuquerque doctors will eventually say, "We're sorry, but we've done all we can." And I'll feel sick and sad and guilty all over again, but this time it will be for someone who literally held my hand through this process. It won't make sense that someone so tough and kind at the same time doesn't live, but that I get to. I will never get it. I will never know why I was spared.

What I do get right now is how she's feeling about the new port and the new treatment. My heart breaks for her. I don't know what I would do if Dr. C found new spots this time around. Little Nolan sleeping in the next room is my motivation for staying well these days, along with the promise of seeing Johanna finish grad school and helping Zach and Lesley move into their first real home. I want to be well. I want to be well for the rest of my life.

I go to Love Field with Johanna, Nolan in the car seat in the back. I get out and hug her and stick my head in and kiss Nolan. The entire time, I'm praying to myself, *No cancer, no cancer, no cancer.* It may be selfish praying only for myself and no one else, but I think I've earned selfish for a minute.

I've booked a room at the Holiday Inn near Reliant Park. I forget each time how weird it is to stay near the Texas Medical Center. There are patients everywhere, identifiable either by the medical center bracelets they all wear, or by their wigs and walkers and wheelchairs in the hotel lobby. There are people like me, looking like they're doing fine, but underneath, we're all in the same boat. We either are now or have been significantly ill, and we're just getting by, doing the best we can, treading water until we get either the good news or the bad news. We'll either sink or swim.

Coming alone was a bad idea, I think. A really bad idea. I need someone to share these thoughts with. I need Johanna by my side, bossing me into giving her the room keycard. I always lose mine, so by default, she is always in charge of it. I go into my silent room and look out over the parking lot of Reliant Stadium. I wish I was here for a baseball game, that it was May instead of December. I'm lonely again. Still.

I'm not coming by myself again. I'm dreading the ride in the shuttle over to MD Anderson. My blood test is in a new place, as is my CT scan. If Johanna were here, she'd already have it mapped in her head and on her phone. I'm winging it. I am learning to live without Johanna managing me. She deserves uninterrupted time in grad school. I'm well, dammit!

I have a good book on my Kindle, but I plan to stop in the library for a new paperback. The MD Anderson library is filled with donated books that you can carry out and keep or return as you see fit. Or you can just leave your book on a table in a waiting room, and it will eventually be picked up and returned to the first-floor library. I like all those books lying around, waiting for me or some other cancer patient or caregiver to pick them up and be transported elsewhere, if only in theory.

On the shuttle bus, I ride with a man from Kansas who has staples in a swirl on a bald spot above his right ear. "Yeah, I had a tumor they removed fourteen days ago. Going to get my staples out today," he says.

Fourteen days? He's up and walking around after having a brain tumor removed only fourteen days ago? Wow. On my right side is a man from Saudi Arabia, speaking perfectly clipped English, telling me he has lymphoma. It was cleared up for eighteen months, and he went home to work, but now he's had a recurrence, and he's headed to the Mays Clinic to begin a new round of treatment. "I will live here for the next ninety days," he says simply. "Then maybe, hopefully..." He presses his lips together.

His voice trails off. Yes. Maybe. Hopefully. He says he is pleased to come here, to the best medical facility in the world, and that his wife Skypes him every night, encouraging him while his three children stand behind her. "They wait for their turn to tell me what they did on this day. I always feel better when I see them on the screen." I am selfishly unhappy about being here alone for two days. He will be here alone for ninety days. I want to hug him, but he is so proper. I know it would be a bad move.

This is what I had forgotten about MD Anderson: there are so many sick people here. Waiting to get on the elevator. Waiting outside for their shuttle to arrive. In the cafeteria. They make me feel proud and brave, and at the same time they make me feel desperate.

"Oh please, God, don't let me be one of the really sick ones," I pray, and then I'm ashamed because I'm sure I should say something like, "Thy will be done." I'm alternately fascinated and freaked out by this place. I just want to be well. To stay well.

Ironically, Yvette and Jerry are here today as well, trying to get a handle on whether he should have more treatments or surgery for his stubbornly advancing prostate cancer. I would love to see her, but the word is that Jerry is having a hard time with all this, that he's depressed and sad and angry about how things are going. Yvette calls me during my blood test and says, "If you get bad news, I told Jerry I'm By Gawd dropping everything and coming to find you." I'm comforted. My Yvette is somewhere in this crazy complex of buildings, ready to help if I need it.

The CT scan takes hours. I forgot how awful this process is, how you wait in a huge room full of sick people for them to call your name. They never get my name right. They twist Buneesa, my legal name, into Vanessa or Boo-neesa. The first call back is for counseling and to get me started drinking the contrast. I remember that having a CT scan is equivalent to having fifty chest X-rays. That's a lot of radiation. This will be my eleventh CT scan this year. Pair all that with the chemicals I've ingested through my port, and I'm like a walking glow stick. But this is what we do.

I ask for the clear liquid, flavored with Sprite. The first time I had a CT scan here, they gave me the mocha-flavored milky contrast. It was like drinking a bottle of Maalox with a chemical twist and a chocolate coffee chaser. After not eating for all those hours and then drinking that, I left the scan, went back to the room, and threw up for hours, Johanna outside the bathroom with a 7-Up.

The next time, I tried the clear liquid, and when they offered flavors, I chose cranberry, forgetting that cranberry juice gives me heartburn. I spent another several hours in misery.

So now I ask for clear liquid flavored with Sprite. The counselor explains that I will have three types of infusions — the contrast I'm drinking, the IV contrast, and the anal contrast.

"Whoa, whoa, whoa! Wait a minute. What do you mean by anal contrast?" I say.

"Let me check the orders." She types rapidly on her keyboard. "Yes, Dr. C has ordered an anal contrast. That simply means that the tech will insert a tube into your rectum, and contrast will be introduced in that manner."

Honestly? This process is not difficult enough without an added tube in my rectum? Do they know that I sometimes have issues with that part of my body, that I don't need any foreign objects inserted to make it worse? I am exhausted with worrying and thinking about the results. Now I have to think about a tube in my rectum and a possible accident?

This is a new challenge in my life. I never know when sudden, violent diarrhea will jump into the mix. I'm on a Stage IV Colon Cancer Facebook page, and we all discuss how this is just one of the special side effects of having so much of my colon removed. I am dehydrated all the time because they removed the part that absorbs liquid, and I have a lot of diarrhea. It is my new normal. A tube in my rectum is not a welcome thought.

I decide to say the Martin prayer and just ask God to put blinders on me.

CT scan with anal contrast. The good news is that I no longer have to have the high-speed heavy dose of contrast into my liver. This time, they're looking from my chest to my pelvis because evidently, the next place colon cancer metastasizes after your liver is the lungs. I didn't know this in the beginning, but now I have a couple more organs to be anxious about. My lungs could be next, like Sarah's. Or my brain.

Here is what I'm learning about cancer: the anxiety will never completely go away. The medical procedures will continue forever, or at least for the next five years.

I'm so tired of learning about cancer. I want to be back in the living room in Dallas, holding Nolan. I'm so tired of being afraid. Truly tired. Just when I think the fear is all gone, it comes back.

CHAPTER 50

I'm Grateful

⌁➤

It is Wednesday morning, and I'm in my room at the Holiday Inn Express Houston, dressing to go see Dr. C and hear my follow-up test results. I should have known better than to come here alone. I should have insisted that Belinda come with me, or I should have begged the new guy, although it is way too early in this relationship to do that. We've been seeing each other only sporadically for a month. A trip to the cancer surgeon might be a bit much this early in the game. Just hanging out with someone is a bit much.

Here is something I don't know today: the new guy will be sweet and smart and somewhat attentive for another couple of months until the next time I have to have some sort of scan. He'll offer to take me. And after the scan, I will never see him again. Never. Not a phone call. Just a drop-off at the curb and a curt, "I gotta run home." Five days after the drop-off, there will be an email with an explanation that I'm impossible to get along with. There will never be another call or text or explanation. I'll be certain that my having to have cancer scans will be the issue. But I'll never know. Either cancer or my craziness will kill the most marginal of relationships.

It could certainly be my craziness. But a month or two after that guy disappears, I will also have a meet and greet from an online dating service. I'll meet the guy — someone who works for the City in a rather official capacity — at Second Street in the Railyard for a beer and we will eventually get to the cancer conversation. I'll go to the restroom and come back to the table to find that he's disappeared. Leaving me with the check. Call me crazy, but the cancer might just be a date killer.

But right now, it is December, and I'm in Houston. I didn't sleep a wink last night. I lay awake in my bed, thinking about the cancer returning, about the stitch in my side that I've been trying to ignore for the past couple of weeks. I think about my aching bones, which someone in my Facebook cancer clique says is residue from the chemo. Are these aches and pains real, or have I conjured them up from nowhere? Is the cancer back? Did Dr. C miss a polyp or a glowing spot? Hardly possible, I know, but maybe?

I'm dreading the visit to the clinic but I also can't wait to get this over with. I realize that my entire cancer journey has been like this, feeling one way one minute, followed almost immediately by another feeling that is an exact contradiction of the first. I've been jerked around emotionally for the past year.

I shower and put on my little brown dress. I wish I were thinner. In my ongoing shallowness and self-consciousness, I still have a bit of a crush on Dr. C and always want to be the most attractive person he's seeing today. I also want to be the healthiest. I also want to just stay here in the room and watch the *TODAY* show. I exhaust myself with my waffling.

My appointment is early so that I can get to the airport and catch a 1:30 p.m. plane back to Dallas and my kids. I catch the shuttle over to MD Anderson. I don't talk to anyone on this trip. I'm far too nervous, and I'm certain that one word out of my mouth will turn into a sob. I make my way up to the gastro clinic on the seventh floor.

This is all so familiar now. I remember the first time we came, how impressed we were with everything, how awe-inspiring and scary it was to Johanna and me. There are still the lines of pale, sick people waiting for elevators, and I say a silent prayer that I am past that. I stick my head in the first-floor library for old time's sake and grab a fat book about the Civil War.

I hope I'll take this book home and never have to return it because I won't be coming back, at least not for a long time. I hope Dr. C will say everything is perfect, and I'm now free to get on with my life.

I'm called in and have a short consult with Angela, the PA who always sees me first. We hug each other. She feels like family.

"You look amazing," she says, smiling as she turns to my file. "Are you feeling good?"

"I feel like a million bucks, except that I didn't sleep at all last night."

"Scanxiety, right?"

I laugh. "Well, I didn't know the technical term for it, but yeah, I'm a mess."

"I'm going to take down some information, and then I'm going to let Dr. C tell you the good news. But it is really good news."

I immediately start to cry with relief. I had no idea how anxiously I was holding my breath, fearful that the cancer had returned. I know I sometimes feel adrift without the cancer to anchor me to life and without all the people who cheered me to the finish line. But the truth is that having a bad scan would be the absolute worst news in the world.

Angela hands me a tissue. "This is the best part of my job," she says, "seeing people get well and stay well."

She is so young and healthy. I can't imagine what her days are like, but I know that Dr. C has a stellar record of removing tumors and lopping off liver portions and getting rid of cancer. I hope she gets to deliver that smile and immense relief to patients all day long today.

She has me lie on the table, and she looks at my scar. "Wow! Look at how pretty your scar is."

I have only thought of my scar as something ugly, but now I see it through her eyes. I am well, my scar has faded from the ugly red stapled gash it was nine months ago, and I feel good. My scar is not my enemy. It really is pretty.

I get back in my chair, and she ushers Dr. C in. He gives me a bear hug, laughs with delight at seeing me, and tells me the same thing Angela did.

"You look great, Bunny. So much better than the first time I met you."

I tingle with pleasure from his kind words, and I know they aren't manufactured. I was sad and unhealthy when I first came here. I had just had my sixth chemo treatment and I was beat up. My hair was starting to thin, and the steroids were puffing me up. I was pale, and I had spent far too many days on the red couch, plugged into marginal TV.

"I feel great, thanks to you," I respond.

He smiles. "Nah, you did most of this yourself. I just helped you along and got the ugly stuff out of your system."

I am crying again. I am an emotional mess, and he takes this chance to tell me that the scans were clear, that there is absolutely no evidence of disease. He goes on to say that he and Angela are moving across the street to Baylor Medical Center, that he'll be the head of the Baylor Oncology Surgical Team or something like that, and that I'm welcome to follow them there.

"I'd follow you anywhere, Doc. If you moved your practice to Alaska, I'd figure out how to continue to see you."

"Now that's what I like to hear."

We continue to visit about his last trip to Albuquerque to see his mom, about green chile, and about snow skiing, which I haven't done since my diagnosis.

"It's time to get back on the slopes," he says. I think about how it's time to get back to doing something I love. The holidays are coming, and Johanna is moving back to New Mexico after this semester, going to grad school in Albuquerque. It's time to have some fun and stop moping.

When we are almost done, he extracts a promise from me that I'll do something especially nice for myself to celebrate. I promise and regretfully leave the clinic. Nothing feels quite like hearing those words from that man, and I want to linger over them. If I follow him to Baylor, I won't have a reason to ever return to MD Anderson unless, heaven forbid, some family member has to be here. I know that if anyone I know has a cancer scare, I'm going to advise them to get here immediately. These people know what they're doing. MD Anderson is the number one cancer treatment center in the United States. While I was happy with the treatment I got at home, I know I'd now come here immediately just to get the expert second opinion.

I am starving now that my nerves have settled down. I go downstairs, sit with the crowd in the cafeteria, and eat steak and eggs and grits. I don't care what I weigh right now. I am going to eat exactly what I want on this day to celebrate my good fortune.

After the breakfast among people who are still being treated, the families waiting for news from a surgeon, the balding women, and the men on canes and walkers, after feeling guilty for being in such good health, I find my way to the chapel. It's just down the hall from the cafeteria, and I've seen the entrance many times. Now I want to be there. I want to say thanks.

I sit quietly for a minute. There are two other women in the room, and they both have their heads bowed. One shakes her head back and forth, and I can tell she is sobbing. My heart goes out to her for whatever miracle she's seeking. I ask God to bless her in whatever way she needs.

"Thank you, thank you, thank you," I say over and over. "Thank you for Johanna and Zachary and Lesley and Nolan, who got me through this. Thank you for my parents, who prayed every minute of every day while they worried themselves almost sick over me. Thank you for all the people out there who gave me their love and care. Thank you for Dr. L and the nurses at the chemo suite. Thank you for Angela and Dr. C. Thank you, thank you, thank you."

I cry a lot, and then I go outside and wait for my shuttle to show up. I take a picture of the lush botanical gardens across the street and post it on Facebook, saying I think it's beautiful, but I'm relieved that I don't have to come back here anymore. My next follow-up will be in Santa Fe. I've promised Dr. C that I'll come back once a year for a follow-up with him, but that will be at Baylor. And it will all be fine.

I am headed to my hotel, where I'll pack and get a cab to the airport. I call my list of people to pass along the news—Johanna first, then Mom, Zach, T. J., Sabrina, Glena, Shelley, Yvette, Jennifer, Jeanne. After I get through security at the Houston airport, I head to Pappadeaux, where I order a dozen oysters on the half shell as part of the ongoing celebration of the day. I am beyond happy. I feel like I'm floating.

I don't need my red notebook right now. The gratitude is everywhere. My heart is full of it.

CHAPTER 51

My Goliath

⁀→

It's Christmas Eve, and I'm sitting in the 9:00 p.m. service at Christ Church Santa Fe. I am surrounded by my people, mostly those from the Wine-Drinking Bible Study Group. Mari Anne sits on my left. Sweet Asha and her husband sit in front of me to the right, with their daughters at the end of the row. Kristi and Lee are in the front row ahead of me, with her mom, Doris, my cancer and surgery pal, and their daughter, Logan. Kristi's little Raylee and Ryan are in the church commons area, waiting to come onstage as Violet and a Woodstock in *A Charlie Brown Christmas*.

Austin Ban sits next to Mari Anne on the other side, and Martin sits at the end of our row. Across the aisle are three friends from our Bible study group. Johanna is in the commons, herding the baby Woodstocks. Jennifer is backstage with the costume designer, but in a minute, she'll join Drew and her boys three rows behind me.

These are some of the people I love best in Santa Fe. I am exhausted yet exuberant. We have been at this for months, and today we've been at it since 3:00 p.m., doing makeup, putting costumes on kids, running back and forth from the children's classrooms to the stage with the Woodstocks, and helping with the meal Christ Church has brought in for the cast and crew.

The crowd at this service is small compared to the earlier performance at 5:00 p.m. In that service, we ran out of the 650 playbills and bulletins we printed last week. We had to get chairs out of the commons, and even with all the extra seating, people were standing against the back wall. Rick, the sexton, estimates we had more than 600 people in our sanctuary, which seats 480 at full capacity. It seems all of Santa Fe showed up to share Christmas Eve with us.

After months of planning, practicing, creating costumes and stage sets, going over lines with kids, and teaching three-year-olds to walk across the stage carrying signs in their bright yellow Woodstock costumes, we are done. Except for this last performance of *A Charlie Brown Christmas* by the children of Christ Church, all the work is over.

In August, I got an email from Jennifer, asking for prayer. She wanted to make the children's ministry more effective. She wanted the kids in the program, who range from babies through junior high, to feel God's love more fully. She said she needed prayer because she also needed to recruit more help, and she really wanted people who felt led to be a part of the ministry. I volunteered. At the time I needed inspiration and she needed help. It felt like a good trade, especially given the months she spent in doctor's offices with me.

At first, I taught Gospel Journey once a month during children's church. I was awkward with the kids in the beginning, knowing I was a nerdy old lady to most of them. It felt to me like we were mostly trying to use up time, but on occasion, I'd ask a question, and a tiny sliver of God's light would shine through in their bright faces and raised hands.

One lesson I taught was on David and Goliath. I brought a roll of duct tape and a tape measure to the class. "Who knows how to use one of these?" I asked, holding up the tape measure. Josiah, Evan, and Hardie leapt to their feet and I had them measure a length of nine feet on the floor, marking each end with the duct tape.

"Okay, I need Johnnie and Will to lie down between these marks." Lauren's two boys lay end to end and didn't reach the marks. Evan suggested that he take five-year-old Will's place, and after much wrangling and squirming, we came up with two bodies that equaled nine feet.

"So, Goliath was about as big as Evan and Johnnie would be if Johnnie stood on Evan's shoulders." Their eyes were as big as saucers. "And David was probably as big as Josiah all by himself." I had filled little bags with five smooth stones and handed those around, knowing that touching, feeling, and seeing are a hundred times more effective than just hearing. It was an ambitious undertaking, passing around bags of rocks in a classroom with elementary-school boys, but they were all eager to hold and touch the stones and think of one of those little stones knocking down a brute like Goliath.

When I asked how in the world David could have been so brave to face Goliath, Johnny Grassmick yelled, "Because he had Jesus to help him!" The other kids raised their fists and said, "*Yeah!*" like they had just reached a new level on their Nintendo DS. I said a silent prayer of thanksgiving. Maybe one of them would one day remember this very moment. Maybe not, but I knew I would.

It dawned on me that I had faced my own Goliath, and with God's help and that of a lot of people who loved me, I had defeated it. I also knew the red notebook had kept me awake and aware of the possibility that the cancer might not be the winner of this battle. I don't know the exact formula that got me to this place, but I know I didn't conjure up healing all on my own. That it wasn't just the chemo and surgery.

So working with the children hadn't been about the children at all. It had been about me as well. I had needed that moment to remember what my life was all about. That, in

Johnny Grassmick's second-grade wisdom, any giant I faced could most likely be defeated if I had the right combination of grace and love and gratitude to help me.

Here we are now, on Christmas Eve, in a quiet church, waiting for the second performance to begin. The jazz trio begins running through the opening measures. Jonah as Charlie Brown and Gabe as Linus walk down the aisle with their beginning lines, and we are off and running. This performance is better than the earlier one, and we are all more relaxed. Mari Anne leans over and squeezes my hand. I send up a silent prayer of gratitude for her, for this privilege of sitting with her. Snoopy wanders out from the wings, nine little Woodstocks following, all of them a bit sleepy to be up this late, one with his cowboy boots showing under his costume, but still as cute as the first day we tried those bright yellow costumes on them.

And the story begins.

After all the lines have been hit perfectly, after the set changes have happened without a hitch, after Linus has quoted the Christmas story from Luke 2 without missing a beat, after the cast has sung "Hark the Herald Angels Sing" with little Emma leading them in her clear voice, after the bows and the standing ovation, Martin gets up to give us a short reflection on the Gospel and Charlie Brown. He talks about how the shepherds who were the very first people to find Christ were really the fringe of society. He likens them to Jesse from *Breaking Bad*. "They were sort of the misfits, the bad boys of society, those shepherds. They weren't religious leaders. They were the guys who couldn't find jobs anywhere else. They were the kids who stayed up all night and slept all day. But God chose them to be the very first members of society to have contact with the Christ child."

This is what frequently happens with Martin. You think he's going to tell you a standard story from the Bible and make it make more sense to you. But then he gives it a twist. He talks about how the televised version of *A Charlie Brown Christmas* almost didn't get onto CBS, about how having Linus read from the King James Version Bible was considered a huge commercial risk, but how afterward, it was considered a seminal moment in television history.

After Martin speaks in his quiet, inspiring Martin voice, helping us to be grateful that we're all God's misfits, but He loves us anyway, we stand and sing several carols. We go forward for communion, and we all sing "Joy to the World." While we're singing, several members go forward and light candles from the advent candle. They circulate through the crowd, lighting the small candles we were handed at the beginning of the service.

At the moment our candles are all lit, the lights dim, and we begin singing "Silent Night," standing in the glow of our own candlelight. It is late, and I'm tired. Johanna has come in from herding the Woodstocks on stage and sits behind me. At some point during Martin's talk, Mari Anne got up to check on things backstage, and now she returns and sits with Johanna. I have Austin Ban and four-year-old Ryan Hunt, out of his Woodstock costume, next to me. Austin helps Ryan get his candle lit. I am somehow magically surrounded by people I love and who love me back, unconditionally. People whose love helped me get well.

I watch little Ryan's face, his blue eyes shining, as we begin to sing "Silent Night," and I am overcome with an odd mixture of love and happiness, something so big and full that I almost can't bear it. Of course, I cry, just because I tend to do that a lot. Mostly I look around me, at all these people who have prayed for me, brought me meals, and held my hand. I look at Ryan and his sweet face and at Austin bending down to make sure he can manage the lit candle. I look at Johanna in the row behind me, singing and holding Mari Anne's hand. Then I look at the window above the pulpit, where I can see stars in the dark sky. "All is calm, all is bright…" we sing, and I realize that the odd mixture in my heart is grace. And hope. Anna Lamott says that grace is a mystery, that it finds us where we are, but it doesn't leave us there, that it takes us to a new place. That's what I feel. That I've been touched by something much bigger than my life and taken to a new place where I am healthy and well and where there's nothing but hope.

As we finish singing and blow out our candles, there is a moment of silence. In that moment, I say thank you one more time.

CHAPTER 52

What Now?

⌁➤

I had a magical Christmas Eve in Santa Fe and Christmas Day in Logan with my parents and Zach, Lesley, and Nolan, who was a beautiful, chubby, almost-nine-month-old, snuggly baby. I had New Year's Eve at Sabrina and Bruce's with all her cousins and New Guy, who is sometimes fun and sometimes not-so-much-fun and cranky, but with whom I'm trying to be as normal as possible. After all those months of wishing I had someone in my life, I'm finding that his presence is frequently chafing, like a pair of too tight shoes. The worst thing about this relationship is that he is clearly sick to death of hearing about the cancer, the cancer, the cancer. The people who have been with me through all of it want to talk about it and congratulate me and hear how I'm feeling.

He withdraws during those conversations. I have a bad gut feeling about that part. I don't know yet that my bad gut will be proven right eventually. It's an interesting dynamic. Am I once again spending time with the wrong guy? Of course, the answer is yes, but I'll have to wait until my next scan to know that he's going to dump me.

Johanna and my family and friends have all been in the middle of my being diagnosed, struggling through treatment and surgery and getting well. They celebrate every milestone. New Guy seems to be standing on the sidelines, shaking his head, like someone who walked in on the last quarter of a basketball game that's not very compelling, where the score is obviously in my favor. Why all the hullabaloo? Why do we have to keep beating this dead horse?

Jeanne comes to town and insists on taking me out for a celebration dinner, wanting to commemorate my being completely well. I can tell from his comments about her enthusiasm that he doesn't quite get it.

But what should I expect? He wasn't here in the trenches. He frequently says all the right things. He's just not on the cancer bandwagon. Not his thing.

But he is not at the center of my universe. At the center is my compulsion to *do something*. I am certain that I was spared for a reason and that I got through 2012 and the Last Boyfriend debacle and my move to Santa Fe and my cancer diagnosis for a reason. There is something else. I just need to find it, and now that I'm feeling physically well, it must be about to make itself evident.

What am I supposed to be doing?

I continue to work for my clients, writing website content and blogs and working their social media platforms like a crazy woman. It is a sweet gig, but it's also a bit isolating. Other than a meeting here and there outside the house, or a trip to Austin to meet with the birthing center staff on occasion, I'm alone. A lot.

It makes for a lot of surfing the web when I should be working, writing, typing in a status for Skyland Aircraft, or posting a food photo for The Ranch House. I've hooked myself up with a list of colon cancer groups on Twitter with names like Colon Cancer Alliance, Chris4Life, Colontown, and Fight Colorectal Cancer. I move restlessly back and forth between the birthing center Twitter account and my own, going to TweetDeck to schedule posts, and then reading tweets from everyone I'm following.

It's January and I'm still trying to make sense of my cancer diagnosis. Maybe "make sense" is not the right phrase. Maybe I'm still trying to find my way out of it. I seem to be having a hard time with that. I feel like I've stalled somewhere. I don't know what to do with myself. I should be celebrating on a daily basis, but instead, I'm feeling flat. I still write in the red notebook, which has been replaced by a small blue spiral notebook. I write nondescript things like, *My health, my family, my Santa Fe life, my faith.*

What did it all mean? What now? I want to wrap it up, put it into a nice little box, make sense of it, and move on with my life. I want an ending that is inspiring, but I can't find it. Maybe simply surviving is inspiring enough. But it doesn't feel quite like enough. Everyone else may feel inspired; I just feel like nothing.

I get on Twitter one day late in January, as I always do to post for one of my clients, and I decide to check out the list of cancer information outlets I've started following. One has a tweet that says, "Don't forget! This Wednesday is the last day to apply for a Call on Congress scholarship #FCRC."

FCRC stands for Fight Colorectal Cancer. I don't love the name, but at least it is very clear about what the organization is and what it does. I also have no idea what "Call on Congress" means, but it sounds like something fun might be about to happen in D.C. I can fill out an application, can't I? I'm sure I won't be chosen because I have no idea what the organization really does or what Call on Congress is, but why not give it a shot?

The form is on a link on FCRC's website, which I explore for a minute. I'm so accomplished at exploring websites about cancer. I'm also so sick of exploring websites about cancer.

I go to the FCRC Facebook page, where there are images of people on the steps of the Capitol, all wearing white shirts with bright blue letters that bear the name of the organization.

They're smiling and raising strong arms to show off their biceps. It looks like a fighting stance. This looks like a group I could have some fun with.

I go to the scholarship form and fill it out. I have the impression that Call on Congress is some sort of gathering where the group will lobby for something vaguely colon cancer-ish. I think the name of the organization is a little daunting—Fight Colorectal Cancer? The addition of the rectal part sounds icky to me. Yes, I know we need to openly talk about our rectums, but are you really going to win friends and influence people with a name like that?

No matter. I'm going to apply for the fun of it. I have no expectation of winning a spot on the team, but I'm starting to think I'd like to get more personally involved with groups that are trying to fight cancer. I'm far enough out from my diagnosis to want to make a difference for someone else. Just posting on my personal Facebook page on a regular basis that everyone *must get scanned now* isn't enough. I want to fight. I want to get in on the war against colon cancer. I don't know if Fight Colorectal Cancer is my group, but I'll give it a shot.

My application tells the story about my stage IV diagnosis and my subsequent treatment. I add that I'm politically active and that because New Mexico is such a small state, I'm actually acquainted with a couple of my senators and representatives. I say that Congresswoman Michelle Lujan Grisham and I used to be close friends. I'll be happy to stop by her office and say hello if that's part of the protocol.

Fight Colorectal Cancer describes itself as an advocacy group, and while I'm uncertain what that means, it is touted as a top-rated cancer nonprofit. I submit my application and don't consider it again. I'll try again next year, when I know even more about the group.

On a Wednesday early in February, I get an email from someone named Emily White. It reads, "Congratulations! You have been chosen to receive a scholarship to attend Call on Congress on March 16–19 in Washington, D.C." It goes on to state that my airfare and room and board will be covered as part of the scholarship. I'll be expected to spend two days training and a day on Capitol Hill, meeting with my congressional delegation to discuss issues facing colorectal cancer patients.

I am stunned. I had no idea that I even had a chance at this. I call Johanna immediately, and she's as thrilled as I am. It takes us only about two minutes to realize that she has a flight voucher and could go along with me for a visit to D.C. If I could afford hotel rooms for a few days ahead of time, this trip could be a bit of a reward for her caretaking.

I get on Facebook and message my first college roommate, Claire, who lives in McLean, Virginia, just outside D.C. A plan is hatched. Johanna and I will go to D.C. a few days early, sightsee and stay with Claire, and then I'll do the FCRC Call on Congress.

I have something to do. I'm headed to D.C. I have a cause!

CHAPTER 53

I Have a Cause

⌒⤳

It's Sunday morning in Washington, D.C., and Johanna just left in a cab to go to the airport. She's headed home to New Mexico. I'm in a panic. After weeks of anticipation, I'm here. We've had four days at my old college roommate Claire's house, treating Johanna to a much-deserved vacation of sightseeing, good food, visiting with old friends, staying up late to talk about college days with Claire, sitting on the steps of memorials, and gazing down the mall at the Capitol building. Once again, Johanna and I have had a great time together.

But now, I'm all alone in a room at the Westin Alexandria with a stranger, a girl named Heather from some Midwestern state that I can't quite remember. I'm exhausted. I hardly slept last night, thinking about today, about getting out there and meeting everyone from Fight Colorectal Cancer. Who do I think I am? What do I have to say? And why am I so scared?

This is exactly what I wanted to do. I wanted to find a cause, and I wanted to give my energy to it. Instead, I find myself cowering in the shower, wondering if I brought the right clothes. I'm pretty sure I didn't.

The Wine-Drinking Bible Study Girls really came through on the jewelry front. I sent out a prayer request for safe travels and a productive trip, along with a request for any authentic Southwestern jewelry they might have. I also needed luggage.

I have no nice luggage, just an oilcloth bag from Mexico in which I tote around my weekend stuff when I travel, which is inappropriate for air travel.

Lauren showed up with a Ralph Lauren suitcase and a turquoise squash blossom necklace, the type I've coveted my entire life. "Ryan gave this to me as an anniversary present. He'll kill me if it gets lost," she said, giving me a hug, trusting me with something she treasures.

"I'll guard it with my life. And thanks. Love it!"

Mari Anne dug in her purse last Sunday at church and produced drop turquoise earrings and a bracelet. "These were Christmas gifts from Martin and the kids," she said, "Wear them well."

Kelly offered an antique Navajo necklace, but when she said she needed to get into the safe to retrieve it, I held up my hand. "No way," I said, thinking that I was already anxious about Lauren's squash blossom and Mar's bracelet. "But thanks for offering."

Megan met me at the post office downtown with a bag. "Here's a great silver necklace," she said, reaching in the bag and pulling out a red box. "Roy bought it from a designer here in town. Oh, and here's a really cool shawl. Maybe it will go with your celebration dinner dress."

The "shawl" was a woven piece of gossamer so fine it felt like a spider's web, a beautiful deep blue and gray spider's web. "Wow, Megan," was all I could say, and she waved my response away.

"Just wear it and have fun," she said, smiling at me. "This is such an amazing thing you're doing. We are all so proud of you."

That's what I'm getting from people. They seem to see my coming to D.C. as a great sacrifice on my part, and they're applauding my efforts. I don't see it that way at all. I'm getting a free trip, and I might get to meet my congressional delegation, and I just might make the tiniest difference in the direction colon cancer research will take in the next decade. Or I might just be petrified by fear, like I am right now.

Last night, Johanna and I had dinner with my roommate and a woman from Wyoming or Montana. She asked me what my story was, and I said, "Oh, I had a little bit of stage IV colon cancer with mets to my liver. But I'm well now."

The cancer community knows that "mets" is short for metastasis, the place where my cancer landed other than my colon, the condition that qualifies mine as stage IV. I've learned that there's a hierarchy in cancer, where your status among survivors is determined by where your "mets" are. I'll learn that liver mets are not nearly as impressive as lung mets, and that brain mets plus survival get you the widest stares. Right now, I'm not feeling very impressive. I feel like I'm the uncool kid in high school.

The Wyoming/Montana girl looked at me with her wide, blue eyes. "So are you saying you're in remission or just NED?"

I know enough to know that NED means "No Evidence of Disease." It seems to be a catchphrase for "I think I'm well, and there's no evidence that I have cancer, but it could reappear at any minute." At least, that's what my inexperienced mind hears.

"Well, my doctor says I'm cancer-free," I say, looking at Johanna helplessly. I *am* cancer-free. Or so I thought.

"Yeah, her doctor says it's all gone," Johanna says, just the tiniest bit defensively. We are so certain that I'm cancer-free. Doesn't the rest of the world agree with us?

"Hmm," Wyoming/Montana girl says, and I know I've just failed some sort of test in which I'm supposed to know with certainty what my cancer status is.

Then she launches into her cancer story, which involves years of radiation, botched surgeries, ostomy bags, and blockages.

My roommate seems to sense my distress. "Let me tell you my story," she says, in her fresh-faced, sweet way, gently interrupting her friend's sad story of being sick for years. Her husband, who was in his mid-thirties when diagnosed, had just a bit of gastro distress. Then he had a colonoscopy, during which hundreds of polyps were found. "He was diagnosed with Lynch syndrome," she says. I don't know much about Lynch at this point, but I know it has something to do with genetic tendencies, and it isn't good. My MD Anderson tests and subsequent genetic counseling ruled out Lynch on my part.

Heather tells me her Lynch story, the fear that went along with having a very sick husband who chose to have his entire colon removed due to the Lynch. "He won't agree to have our kids tested yet," she says, and I get that she is distressed about this decision. "I just want us to know what we're facing, but he feels guilty that he might have passed it along."

Damn cancer. It is so daunting and so random and so ruthless. I feel a bit more charitable toward my other dinner partner. She didn't choose to be someone who had bad medical care before she got good care. She didn't choose to have cancer. No one gets to choose.

The next morning, my roommate and I head out on King Street to get breakfast, two strangers thrown together in the oddest manner possible. It is bitterly cold in D.C. There's a forecast of yet another big snowstorm for tomorrow. I wonder for the hundredth time what the hell I am doing here.

We get back to the room, and I put on something purple, which I've discovered is the color of cancer survivors. I don't know that I'll stick out like a sore thumb, that everyone in the room will be wearing deep cobalt blue, which is the color of colon cancer.

I find myself in a meeting room with seventy-five or eighty other people. Most of them are greeting one another with shouts and hugs. This is a crowd that knows each other well. We've been given name tags and notebooks in the hall outside, and there are ribbons to attach to the tag that say "Survivor" or "Caregiver" or "Patient." I get the Survivor tag, which turns out to have some cache in this group. Several people ask me my story or my stage, and I am learning to quickly say, "I had stage four with mets to my liver. I'm almost a year out from my surgery. Cancer-free these days."

"Good for you," someone says in response, and they are on to the next person. Everyone is friendly but busy.

There's a panel of presenters. They talk about current research and the Affordable Care Act. I'm hoping this is not what the entire day will be about because I didn't sleep at all last night. I'm certain to nod off.

Next there is a father/daughter team at the podium, and he begins to tell their story. He was diagnosed early in February a couple of years ago, "a stubborn old goat of a guy who wouldn't get a colonoscopy, that's who I was." He has a compelling story, and we are laughing at his stubbornness and boneheaded attitude toward his own health. I like this guy. But then he turns to his daughter and says, "And I would have laughed in the face of cancer had it not also decided to attack my baby girl here." In the midst of his treatment, she began to have symptoms that were troubling: oddly shaped stools, stomach pain, blood in her stool.

She tells her own story of the trials associated with doctors who remain convinced that colon cancer is an old man's disease. "I kept telling my doc I wanted a colonoscopy, and he kept patting me on the head, saying I was too young, not to worry, that I probably had irritable bowel syndrome."

The patronizing doc was wrong, and by the time she had a scan, she had stage III colon cancer and needed immediate surgery for a potential blockage. She and her dad alternate telling the story, and there is a screen with photos behind them, showing the two of them in different stages of illness, in hospital beds, hooked up to chemo drips. There is a lot of talk of faith and trial drugs.

We are all crying.

And then comes the good news, that he is cancer-free and that she is currently NED and having frequent scans and tests to be sure there is no recurrence. Everyone stands and cheers.

They sit down, and Emily, the facilitator in charge of the program, takes the mic. "Now it's time for you to tell your story. We'll pass the mic around the room and let you say a few words about why you're here, what your role is, when you were diagnosed if you're a survivor, that sort of thing."

I am floored. And sweating. I don't want to tell my story to this room full of strangers. Until today, I've been the cancer rock star, first as a patient and then as a survivor with cancer ass-kicking superpowers. Now I'm just a face in the crowd, and I'm petrified. I never get petrified. Why the hell did I think I could do this? Who do I think I am?

The stories start. One guy has Lynch syndrome, and his teen son is with him. He points to his boy, "We just had James tested. And he is..." He draws out the answer to add suspense and then shouts, "*negative!*" The room erupts in applause. This guy is obviously an old hand at Call on Congress. Everyone seems to know him, and they are all clapping and smiling. A few get up and go to them both, hugging them.

There are a lot of stories. People cry. Some speak very softly. "I will be on chemo for the rest of my life," a sweet blonde whom I will later know as Belle says. "But my kids are out there in the hallway, and whatever it takes to stay alive for them, I'll do."

The mic moves around the room, and as it gets closer to me, I am completely blank. What exactly *is* my story? Why do I think I have anything to contribute to this gathering?

And then the mic is in my hand. I stand and face the tables of people wearing bright blue. I am shaking.

"Hi. My name is Bunny Terry, and I'm a survivor." It feels like something you'd say at an A.A. meeting, but once the words are out, I'm very close to tears. "I was diagnosed with stage four colon cancer with mets to my liver after only one day of symptoms. I had chemo and surgery at MD Anderson, and more chemo, and I am now cancer-free!" I say it all in a rush, and then I am crying, and the girl sitting next to me stands up to hug me, and I sit down. I don't know why I'm crying, but there is power in this room with these people who all know exactly what has happened to me. I'm not the only rock star anymore, but I am surrounded by so much positive energy that I think I could probably fly if I lifted my arms and tried to take off.

Someone else down the row stands and says, "I'm like Bunny. I had just one day of pain, and then I was diagnosed with stage four colon cancer. My mets were in my lungs. I'm also cancer-free." She smiles and winks at me.

The storytelling takes a long time, but I'll learn later, when I've been asked to join the Grassroots Action Committee and help plan next year's event, that this is considered an essential part of Call on Congress. Getting the words out prepares us for our meetings with our congressional delegation, where we'll say the same story over and over. And it binds us together.

It is perhaps the hardest thing I've done since hearing the words, "You have stage four colon cancer." But by telling my story and hearing everyone else's, I'm aware of a kind of power and acceptance I didn't know existed. All these people have suffered in unimaginable ways, and the truth is that I have hardly suffered at all. But this isn't about comparison. This is about hearing and healing and knowing and accepting and getting up to fight so that someone else doesn't have to face this bullshit disease alone.

A beautiful blonde woman stands with her husband and teenage daughter flanking her on either side. She begins to tell her story, and the daughter joins in, and they are both crying. The daughter says, "I had to stand by and watch my mom go through treatment and surgery. Hearing that my mom had cancer was the worst moment of my life." But she is hard to understand because she is crying so hard. It is an ugly-cry, brokenhearted and sad. The husband steps around the blonde, whom I will learn is Sheila, and wraps his daughter in his arms. "This is always the hardest part," he says, and I am surprised that this is not the first time they've told this story together. It makes me miss Johanna. I vow to bring her next year.

Before the mic has made the entire circuit through the crowd, I am thinking about next year. When this session began, I was only tired and frightened. But now I know I am doing exactly what I am supposed to be doing.

I'm a cancer advocate — for me and for all the people in this room, and for the ones who can't get here, and the ones who didn't make it. What will follow the storytelling is a short program with a video to honor the FCRC members who have passed in the last year, and there will be open weeping in the crowd. I'm here for those cancer victims. I'm here for Sarah. I'm here for people I don't know who will hear the words "You have stage four colon cancer." Mostly I'm just here, determined to do something that makes a difference.

We have a break after the sessions, and I find my way to the hotel bar, where an entire section is taken up by people wearing deep blue. I'm a bit out of place with my purple, but no one makes me feel uncomfortable. Patti, at the end of the table, opens up her arms and waves me in. "Bunny, right?" she says, and pulls up a chair for me. I'm going to sit down and have a drink with my new friends. The Cancer Clique, Johanna will eventually call them. My uncertainty about my future and my purpose has been wiped away.

I'm a cancer advocate.

CHAPTER 54

Who Do I Think I Am?

◊◊▶

In the next two days, I will attend meetings at the American Society of Clinical Oncology, make dozens of new Cancer Clique friends, and travel to Capitol Hill to meet with my congressional delegation. I'll be a bit intimidated by all the information I receive, all the research studies I hear about, all the tips I get for talking to my senators and representatives. I'll drink blue margaritas in the hotel bar because, you know, we're all about blue at Fight Colorectal Cancer. Blue is the color of colon cancer, just like pink is the color of breast cancer.

I'll have a long conversation with a woman whose mother-in-law had the worst possible bout of rectal cancer years ago. She'll tell me her mother-in-law still won't use the word "rectal," and that we have to break down these barriers, that talking about body parts shouldn't be taboo in any way. We'll share stories, and she'll tell me I'm looking amazing, that she knows I'm well and that my cancer won't be coming back. She'll say she can see it in my eyes, and she'll tell me that my story is my most valuable asset. I'll finally realize that I'm talking to Nancy Roach, the founder of Fight Colorectal Cancer, and that she's headed to the White House the next day for the proclamation-issuing ceremony. March will be declared Colorectal Cancer Month, and an initiative to have 80 percent of all eligible adults screened by 2018 will be created.

I'll learn facts that will be stuck in my head by the time I get on the bus to go to the Capitol. Colorectal cancer is the number two cause of cancer deaths in the United States, just behind lung cancer. More than 150,000 Americans will be diagnosed with it, and more than 50,000 will die from it. This year.

I will learn that this is not an "old white guy's disease," as most of the public thinks. I'll meet kids in their twenties who were diagnosed at seventeen and nineteen. I'll spend an hour in the Sam Rayburn basement visiting with Todd Spurrier, a guy who founded Destination X and who is riding a Ducati across America, determined to photograph five hundred people who were diagnosed before they turned fifty. He wants to reach this goal before he turns fifty. Turns out, Todd's dad died from Lynch, and Todd and all his siblings have it. Todd is missing his colon. "I'm not even a semi-colon," he'll laugh. He's riding a donated Ducati across the country, sleeping on the ground, emptying his colostomy bag in state park restrooms.

I'll go into the offices of my delegation, nervous as a cat, and all alone because I'll be the only person from New Mexico in attendance. I'll first meet with Senator Martin Heinrich's legislative assistant, a woman named Jude, and she'll immediately put me at ease.

"Tell me why you're here," she'll say gently, and I'll launch into my story, talking about the evening at the ER, the pain in my side, the colonoscopy, and the surprise and fear that I felt when I heard the diagnosis. Her eyes will shine with tears, and she'll put her hand on mine.

"How can we help you?" she'll ask, and I'll tell her how desperately we need additional research funding, how the NIH has initiatives for increased awareness and scans, how we need to change Medicare laws so that removal and testing of polyps is covered rather than billed to the low-income patient.

As I'm leaving, I'll turn to her in relief and say, "I was so nervous about coming in here to talk to you. I should have sent a lobbyist."

She'll wave her hand and laugh. "We can't stand lobbyists! In a state as poor as New Mexico, and as sparsely populated, why would anyone ever need to pay someone to show up on their behalf? This is the better way. I'll never forget your face or your story."

I want to sing as I walk down the hall to my meeting with Senator Tom Udall's staff. I did it! I actually went alone into Heinrich's office and asked him to help colon cancer patients. And I was okay. I only cried twice.

Tom Udall's staff is even easier. Lauren Arias is an Albuquerque girl, about the same age as Zachary, and she knows a couple of kids from his Academy class. She knows my "I Love New Mexico" blog, and she gets me a cup of coffee and sits down to visit. This is so easy. When I tell my story, she also gets tears in her eyes and has to wipe them away. She knows someone who didn't survive colon cancer, and this story is very personal to her. She promises the senator's support, but more importantly, she promises to keep me in her prayers. I thank her and then ask her to instead pray for the people still suffering.

Finding my way through the snow on the street over to the Rayburn building after those two meetings is like skipping through a park. I am so fired up, and I still have Ben Ray Lujan to visit. I'll try to fit in Michelle Lujan Grisham's office, even though she's not my representative. Michelle and I were friends a long time ago, and I am determined to stick my head in and at least say hello. I want support for this cause anywhere I can find it.

I run into the California girls, who are lugging a box full of information folders around. Erika sighs in frustration.

"We have so many of these to drop off. I don't know how we'll ever make it to everyone's offices."

"Let me have a pile," I say. I am so energized. I want a meeting with every single senator and representative in the country. I'm happy to drop in.

The fear from Saturday and Sunday is gone. The intimidation about meeting with my delegation has disappeared. The paralyzing fear about telling my story aloud to a roomful of strangers is gone. It is true that there is great power in my story, and I can't wait to share it with someone else.

We spend the day on the Hill and find our way back to Alexandria by way of the Metro, dribbling in throughout the afternoon. I ride with Belle and her kids. I am in awe of her strength in the midst of knowing she has to go home and have chemo next week.

There is a celebration dinner tonight, and I consider taking a nap before I groom. I've brought my best dress, the gray confection that I wore to Zach and Lesley's wedding. I'll wear it with the gossamer woven scarf and heavy silver necklace that Megan loaned me.

But I can't nap. I'm still riding high on the events of the day. I meet ten or fifteen other FCRC advocates in the bar, and we are all hugging and talking at once, euphoric after our day on the Hill talking about cancer. I look down my row of chairs at Pam and Rose, two women who started with this organization at least a decade ago. Both of them have ostomies, and Rose also has another bag for her bladder. They are beautiful and healthy, despite their ongoing health issues. Last night, Rose stopped me in the bathroom of the restaurant where twenty of us had gathered and said, "I keep seeing you around. What's your story?"

I was still in the intimidated stage, and I knew she was the head cheerleader for FCRC. I felt like the new kid at school who wasn't really cool enough to be here. I rattled off my story, and she smiled.

"You look amazing. I'm so proud of you for coming here!" She hugged me. "We're going to be great friends."

Now she and Pam were talking hard and fast. Pam, a Southern belle brunette from West Virginia, is waving her arms at her Jersey girl buddy, and they're talking about the upcoming Hausmann Horseshoe Tournament.

"You ever pitch horseshoes, Bunny? I'll bet a girl from New Mexico knows how to throw a ringer or two, don't you?"

"I do. In fact, I think I won a trophy back in the eighties for a Fourth of July horseshoe tournament."

"Well, hon, you're going to have to come on up to New Jersey in July for Rose and Eric's fundraiser. All we do is pitch horseshoes and drink cold beer. And raise money for colon cancer."

The celebration dinner hasn't even begun, but already I know what my life was spared for. It was for this — for sharing my cancer story and making a difference. It was for showing the world that cancer doesn't have to define us or defeat us. That despite all the ugliness and fear and pain, we can claim some sort of victory at the end of the day.

In my room later, before I put on my blue eye shadow and mascara and bright red lipstick, I write in the blue notebook. *Everything, today, everyone — Belle and Todd and Erika and Rose and Eric and Pam and Patti and Heather. Not being afraid. Finally, not being afraid.*

The celebration dinner will be the best part of the trip. There will be dinner and free drinks and dancing, dancing, dancing. Everyone will be on the floor, including Belle, who has now become one of my best pals. I rode on the bus next to her nine-year-old son this morning on our way to the Hill. When I asked him whether he played sports, he very matter-of-factly said, "Nah. When your mom has cancer, you mostly need to be around to help her out." He was not sad or upset or resentful. I knew that Belle had ongoing issues and that she will be on chemo for the rest of her life. In the next several weeks, one treatment will stop working, but she'll hear of a trial that she might be eligible for. She will send out a post on Facebook, asking us all to cross our fingers, wish on stars, and say prayers. On her behalf I will say a lot of desperate prayers.

I also know that she is determined to hang on as long as possible. I agree with her method. If I had that adorable child at home, I'd be fighting every minute for my life. What I don't know is that when I come back in two years, Belle won't be here. She will have lost her battle. Along with Rose the cheerleader. Along with Sarah at home. Along with Randy, the bald guy who sat behind me yesterday in the general information sessions and offered his hand in a very calm greeting, saying to me, "We are so glad you're here to help us."

It's good that we don't know these things in advance. Otherwise, the fight would be too hard.

I was so full of angst about dating and money and being alone and getting well. Now I know that all of that is nothing, that the most important thing I can do with my life and time is this. The rest will fall into place if and when it's supposed to. Making a difference, however small, for someone else who has colon cancer — or any type of cancer for that matter — can't wait. This is exactly where I'm supposed to be.

I sit with my roommate and beautiful, blonde Chris, a thirty-something attorney from Milwaukee. Her roommate, Bonnie from Houston, joins us, and we laugh over our endless glasses of red wine. Chris has just undergone HIPEC surgery, a treatment that included opening her up and spraying her insides with liquid chemo. "This is definitely going to work!" she says victoriously. Chris has two little girls at home, and like Belle, she is determined to stay alive for her babies. Except that she won't. Next year, she'll be another of the faces on the "In Memoriam" video. Thankfully, I don't know that yet.

Kristen from Denver joins us with her curly-headed son, Ben, and we all talk about our day, about this being our victory lap, about next year. Kristen and Bonnie are stage III survivors, still suffering neuropathy in their feet from the brutal chemo treatments they had.

"Ah, what the hell," Kristen says. "I can still dance, even if I can't feel the bottoms of my feet!"

Belle and I dance to ABBA, and the night begins to wear down. At the very end of the evening, the DJ plays Pharell Williams's "Happy," and we empty our seats and stream onto the dance floor. We are happy, crazy happy, and we dance like the little children that some of the Cancer Clique have brought along. There is singing and clapping, and I jitterbug for a second with Nancy Roach before being passed back to my new friend, Chris. We throw our heads back and sing our hearts out.

This is why I was spared. This is why every day I needed to remember what I was grateful for. This is what it was all about. I kicked cancer's ass, and now I plan to help others do the same.

I am happy.

The End

Epilogue

∿➤

"Instructions for living a life. Pay attention.
Be astonished. Tell about it."
Mary Oliver

One of the hardest calls I ever received was when I heard from Will's daughter that Sarah had died. Sarah (not her real name) had been my cancer mentor, and then toward the end of her life, she shut off all communication with everyone other than Will. For the last six months of her life, with the exception of her doctors, she refused to see anyone, saying that she wanted to wait until she got better, that she didn't want anyone to see her looking like a sick person.

Will did it all, the cooking, the cleaning, the bathing, the morphine injections, the caregiving. He will tell you now that all he was able to do was be a witness, that he felt helpless in the face of such physical pain, but that he did the best he could for this strong, stubborn, beautiful woman.

And then one morning he went into the bedroom and she had slipped away in the night, her suffering over and her journey finished. His heart was broken and so was mine.

After that, we spent time together, planning her memorial, gathering photos, creating a video for her service (with the help of Johanna). I kept dropping by pots of green chile stew, trying to get him to eat. I made him go out for pizza with me. I worried that he was going to disappear in his grieving.

Those days, along with our sorrow, and our understanding of one another's life with cancer, developed into something to celebrate. On July 13, 2017, Will and I were married. In all that searching for true love, I never knew that it was right in front of me, that along with all the horrible things cancer might provide, it could also provide amazing gifts.

I knew Will when I was a child, but he was my older brothers' friend, a devastatingly handsome and very cool guy in the 60's. Now he is the same, except that he's in his 60's. I've had a crush on him since I was six years old. It took cancer and the death of someone important to both of us for us to be given this life that seems to be charmed.

Between us we have four children, seven grandsons, and one great-grandson. Life is a gift every day with this man. I still wake every morning and say, "Thank you, thank you, thank you."

I am eight years out from my cancer diagnosis. Will is six years past the loss of Sarah. We learned a lot through our cancer experiences, and we've continued to learn while creating a life together.

Here's what we've learned: That life is precious. That time is short. That remaining grateful is always the answer. That sometimes the only thing you can do is give yourself away. And that to whom much is given, much is required.

Cliches are cliches because they're true. My suggestion is that you never discount these sorts of truths in your life.

Finally, I'll leave you with this, my mantra every day:

If life were any better, I'd have to be two people.

About the Author

∿➤

Bunny Terry is currently the Vice Chair of the Board of the Cancer Foundation for New Mexico, where she is dedicated to helping other cancer patients navigate the treacherous waters of cancer recovery.

In addition to being a fierce advocate for cancer patients, Bunny also runs a successful marketing, speaking, and coaching business and sells residential and farm/ranch property as a broker at Keller Williams Santa Fe.

She lives with her husband in Santa Fe where she is at work on a second book, *Where I Come From*, a collection of essays, mostly true, about the small town on the eastern plains of New Mexico where some of her 64 cousins live. She's also developing *365 Days of Lifesaving Gratitude*, a combination planner and inspiration journal.

Bunny knows everyone has a powerful gratitude story and she would love to hear yours. Feel free to contact her at www.bunnyterry.com

Made in United States
Orlando, FL
16 December 2021

11865336R00157